SOME OF THE THINGS YOU WILL DISCOVER IN THIS LIFE-ENHANCING BOOK

—This program is unique—it is the only one without additional drugs or surgery that has been tested and found to produce improvements in the heart's function.

—How the heart works and what we now know about the effects of diet and stress on the heart.

—Foods to eat and foods to avoid, with over 150 delicious recipes by bestselling cookbook author Martha Rose Shulman.

—An easy-to-follow, illustrated method of stress reduction that takes only minutes a day.

—How you can become more productive while enjoying life more.

Read and enjoy

STRESS, DIET, AND YOUR HEART

DEAN ORNISH, M.D., is currently a Clinical Fellow in Medicine at Harvard Medical School and a resident on the Medical Services of the Massachusetts General Hospital in Boston.

STRESS, DIET, AND YOUR HEART

Dean Ornish, M.D.

With a Foreword by
Alexander Leaf, M.D.

Original Recipes by
Martha Rose Shulman

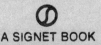

A SIGNET BOOK

NEW AMERICAN LIBRARY

*This book is dedicated
to my teachers, friends, and family.*

NOTE TO THE READER

The ideas, procedures, and suggestions contained in this book are not
intended as a substitute for consulting with your physician. All matters
regarding your health require medical supervision.

I have had dreams, and I have had nightmares.
I overcame the nightmares because of my dreams.

—JONAS SALK, M.D.

Contents

Contents

Acknowledgments

Researching and writing about stress reduction might have been among the most stressful of experiences were it not for the abundance of help I received along the way.

This book represents a collaboration that involved a great number of people. Although I am listed as the sole author, neither the research nor the book would have been possible without the efforts of many others. I would like to acknowledge my gratitude here. Of course, everyone who is acknowledged does not necessarily agree with all of the ideas expressed in the book. The same is true of investigators whose research I have quoted in other chapters.

The major donor to our first cardiovascular research study was the Franzheim Synergy Trust. Kenneth and Susan Franzheim provided me with the opportunity to pursue ideas which at that time were only being formulated. Daniel Dror donated the use of ten rooms at the Plaza Hotel, Houston, to house the patients in our first study. The Woodlands Inn provided accommodations for the initial session at a reduced rate.

Marcia Acciardo, Priscilla Moe, and Eloise Hetherly prepared the meals that we served to the patients during this study. Dr. John Craig provided the illustrations used for the visualization exercises in this study; Dr. Ray Rosenthal helped teach the stress reduction techniques; Dr. Assad Rizk and Marilyn Francis, R.N., supervised the treadmill laboratory, while Drs. Mario Verani and Larry Reduto supervised the nuclear cardiology testing. Most of the patients were referred by Drs. Donald Rochelle and his

Acknowledgments

associates; Frank Rickman, Daniel Jackson, and Richard Jackson referred others.

The major donor to our second cardiovascular research study was Gerald D. Hines. Kevin Alme (president of Leisure Resources Group) donated the use of sixteen two-bedroom condominiums at Horseshoe Bay (near Austin, Texas) to house the patients in this study. Without the generosity of Mr. Hines and Mr. Alme, this work could not have been accomplished. Ron Mitchell allowed the patients to use the recreational facilities of Horseshoe Bay. Joe Elmers of Physio-Controls provided emergency resuscitation equipment, which, fortunately, was not needed. Henry Groppe, Jack Dulworth, and Ralph Frede were instrumental in coordinating support for the study. My parents also have been very generous with their support, for which I am grateful.

The research was also supported by grants from the National Heart and Blood Vessel Research and Demonstration Center, Baylor College of Medicine (HL-1729 from the National Heart, Lung and Blood Institute, National Institutes of Health), and the U.S. Public Health Service Biomedical Research Support Grant (RR-05424-19). Other donors included: the Frank Abraham Student Aid Foundation; Amax Petroleum; Leon and Betty Breton; Norman Cousins; the Fannin Bank; the Kayser Foundation; Merrill Lynch, Inc.; Jeff Montgomery; the Natwin Foundation; the Alvin and Lucy Owsley Foundation; Pennzoil Petroleum; Reed Mining Tools; Mary Rollins; Tom Rollins; Charles Sapp; Seagull Petroleum; Transcontinental Gas Pipe Line Companies; the Holmes Center; Western Equipment, Inc. The grants were administered by Jean King, Ozzie Schoenemann, and Lorraine Harden.

Dr. John Burdine provided the use of his nuclear cardiology laboratory (on very short notice) and allowed us to schedule testing on weekends. Dr. Robert J. Hall gave a weekend of his limited time to supervise the testing and provided advice and critical comments. Drs. Gordon DePuey and Robert Sonnemaker read and interpreted all of the nuclear cardiology studies, and Jim Bietendorf, Gary Myers, and Brad Pounds were the chief technicians. Dr. Paul Baer provided the use of his psychophysiology laboratory, with technical assistance by Allison Fairlie. Mario Nava was technical director of the lipid analyses. Most of the patients were again referred by Dr. Donald Rochelle and his associates; I am also grateful to the other physicians who referred patients.

The project could not have been completed without the other co-investigators in our second study. There is space to list only a fraction of their real contributions. Dr. Larry Scherwitz, the principal co-investigator, was a continual source of ideas and hard work, and he allowed me to share his office during our study. Dr. Shirley Brown worked tirelessly on both the first and the second studies, and she helped edit the recipes in this book. Among other responsibilities, Dr. Sandra McLanahan taught the stress reduction techniques. Dr. Rachelle Doody taught anatomy, physiology, and visualization, developed the idea of having patients draw as an aid to the visualization process, and contributed to the chapter on visualization. Deborah Kesten, M.P.H., taught classes in nutrition education, helped categorize the Five Food Groups, contributed some recipes to the project, and conducted an analysis of the recipes for nutritional adequacy, making modifications in the menus where necessary. Gay McAllister, R.N., provided the Holter monitoring (and moral support) for both the first and second studies. Laverne Dutton, M.S., conducted the Type A interviews and helped in their analysis. Carol Laman also analyzed these interviews for speech characteristics and helped in follow-up data collection. Cathie Haynes, R.N., a cardiovascular nurse specialist, assisted in many aspects of the program. Dr. Jerry Lester conducted a complex and detailed statistical analysis and patiently explained the statistical methods to me. Brother Ron Pickarski contributed some recipe ideas. Carie Seale, LaRhonda Walker, and Patricia Johnson provided valuable secretarial assistance.

Martha Shulman, a gifted cook, planned the menu for the second study, taught cooking classes, and directed food preparation. (Her excellent assistants were Connie Colten and Danny Clark.) She developed the recipes and wrote most of Chapters 14–20. Edith Tagrin and Medical Art at Massachusetts General Hospital drew the illustrations and flow diagrams in Chapter 4 and the hearts in Chapter 11. Medical Illustration at Baylor College of Medicine drew the charts and graphs in the Appendix, except for one provided by Henry V. Brennan of CBS in New York.

Lori Reingold videotaped the first study at the studios of the University of Texas Health Science Center at Houston; Joel

Acknowledgments

Goldblatt and his colleagues at Tele-Techniques videotaped the second study, also on very short notice.

Dr. David Mumford served as mentor, adviser, and confidant during my years at Baylor. Dr. Antonio Gotto provided support and resources to conduct both the first and the second studies at Baylor. Dr. Harold Brown helped guide me through the intricacies of the Human Experimentation Committees. Valuable advice and critical comments at one time or another were also provided by Drs. James K. Alexander, Herbert Benson, Major Bradshaw, William T. Butler, William Castelli, Regis DeSilva, Edgar Haber, Blaine Hollinger, Russ Jaffe, Edward H. Kass, Darwin Labarthe, Bernard Lown, Jim McFarland, Lysle Peterson, Ray Rosenthal, Frank Sacks, George Terrell, Lewis Thomas, Howard K. Thompson, Carlos Vallbona, and Peter Yurchak. Dr. Robert Cameron helped to categorize the hundreds of research articles I'd collected over the years.

The following people offered to donate their valuable time to provide lectures or entertainment for the patients in our second study: The Comedy Workshop (Houston), Norman Cousins, Terry Doody, Keith Harris, Gerald Jampolsky, Ed Lavin, Edgar Mitchell, Marshall Rosenberg, and Stevie Wonder. The American Heart Association and Hartley Productions loaned films to us.

Most of this book was written in New York City on the amazing Wang word processing system, made available to me by the generosity of Joe Ramellini at CBS at the suggestion of Marion Siegel from Wang Laboratories. (Although whatever efficiency was gained by using a word processor was probably lost by its being programmed to play Space Invaders.) The final edit was performed on the Wang system in the Resources and Development Office at Massachusetts General Hospital, courtesy of the generous hearts of Dorothy Newell and Joseph C. Donnelly.

Because the analysis of the research results took much longer than I had anticipated, I had only five weeks to write the book before beginning my internship. I am very grateful to Judith Glassman, who worked with me for five weeks, at least twelve hours a day, almost every day, providing encouragement, organizational ideas, and continual editorial criticisms and suggestions while I was writing this book. She helped transform what would have been a very stressful situation into one that was enjoyable.

I had no plans to write this book until Lester Alexander

Acknowledgments

envisioned it and convinced me that it was feasible and worth doing. I am also grateful to him (and to Richard Smith) for allowing me to sleep in their offices during my five weeks in New York.

I am indebted to all of the following people who took time out from remarkably crowded schedules to read and criticize this book manuscript: Drs. Stephen Calderwood, Phyllis Carr, Anne Goldfeld, John Goodson, Allan Goroll, Stephen Hoffman, Lee Kaplan, Alexander Leaf, Kobi Ledor, Steve Ornish, Doris Platika, Glenn Pransky, Nancy Rigotti, Frank Sacks, Tom Sterne, Donna Phillips, and Andrew Weil. Lester Alexander, Amie Hill, Gini Kopecky, Pamela Morgan, and Karen Thorsen also read the manuscript and provided comments. Philip Mandelkorn and Natalie Ornish made extensive revisions. I am especially grateful to Dr. Leaf for his valuable advice, encouragement, and for writing the Foreword to this book. Special thanks to Dr. George Thibault and John Stoeckle.

It has been a pleasure for me to work with my editor, Jennifer Josephy, and her assistant, Rachel Christmas. Also, it has been a privilege for me to work with and learn from the house staff, physicians, and patients at the Massachusetts General Hospital. Dr. Jim Thomas kindly allowed me to switch internship assignments with him so that I could present the research data at the annual meeting of the American College of Cardiology in April 1982.

I am most indebted for the ideas contained in the research and in this book to S. S. Satchidananda. In many ways, this book is an outgrowth of what I have learned from him. Writing this book helped me to realize just how much he has taught me.

I am grateful for the opportunity to work with the patients who participated in our two research projects. I know that I learned much more from them than they learned from me.

I feel privileged to have been associated with all of the people mentioned; my gratitude to them can never be adequately expressed. I hope that this book allows them to feel that their efforts were in some way worthwhile.

Notes

The program described in the pages that follow is a supplement to—not a replacement for—conventional medical treatments of coronary heart disease. If you have any symptoms to suggest that you may have coronary heart disease (chest tightness or pain, shortness of breath, and so on), see your doctor. While we have documented the short-term benefits of our program in treating coronary heart disease, the long-term effects remain to be studied.

As with any new health program, you would be wise to consult your physician before beginning this one. This is especially true if you are currently taking cardiac medications, since your need for these may be reduced. Of course, any medication changes must be done under your doctor's supervision.

The conclusions of this book are based on a thorough review of the relevant research literature as well as our own studies. However, this book is written primarily for the general public; it is not intended to be a scholarly text. To avoid the distraction of citing hundreds of references, only selected ones are presented for each chapter at the end of the book.

For convenience, I have tended to use masculine pronouns. This is less a reflection of any bias than the fact that most people who have coronary heart disease are men—although the incidence in women is rising. Everything in this book applies equally to women.

For simplicity, the diet and stress management techniques described in this book are referred to as "the program."

Notes

Since most of the ideas presented here interrelate, it has been necessary to repeat some of them at various parts of the text.

The names of the patients have been changed to protect their privacy.

Foreword

Medicine has two traditional functions: to prevent disease from occurring and to cure disease once it has occurred. The major successes of this century have involved both approaches. Better sanitation, housing, nutrition, and immunizations are all measures that have prevented infectious diseases which were the major causes of death in 1900. The introduction and use of antibiotics in the curative mode further reduced mortality from infectious diseases. This two-pronged attack on infections has markedly reduced premature mortality from these traditional scourges of mankind.

The successes in reducing mortality from infections have served to uncover another set of afflictions which now are major causes of disability and death, namely, cardiovascular diseases. Of these, coronary heart disease in our western industrialized world is now the leading cause of death. Medicine has been grappling with this modern killer largely by application of the curative approach: treating established coronary artery disease—angina and nonfatal heart attacks—with a variety of pills and with coronary bypass surgery. This curative approach has proved very expensive, and though it attains some successes, it has one unavoidable inherent limitation. No matter how much we invest in efforts to cure coronary artery disease by surgery or medications, these approaches do not reduce the risk of heart attacks for the next generation. With heart attacks accounting for as many deaths annually in the United States as all other causes of death combined, we are dealing with a modern epidemic still taking a toll of some 600,000 lives per year—despite an encouraging reduction in the death rate in the past two decades. Many of these deaths are sudden, with no suspicion on the part of the victim that he or she was already affected by an advanced state of coronary artery disease. These deaths leave little opportunity for curative medicine to help. Thus the high costs (coronary bypass surgery costs $15,000 to $20,000), the frequency of sudden death, and the failure of curative approaches to reduce the burden of illness in the next generations have all indicated the need to implement preventive measures to reduce the incidence of coronary artery disease.

In the past few years we have been admonished by government and many individual health professionals to accept responsibility for our own health and to adopt healthful living habits. In this book Dr. Dean Ornish provides a very persuasive discussion of the benefits that can accrue to each of us from adopting sensible habits. Though his important research dealt with the beneficial effects of diet and stress reduction upon a group of individuals who had established, serious heart disease, the practices he recommends may be expected to be of even greater value in preventing damage to the heart than in reducing pathology that already exists.

Epidemiologic studies have now revealed the major risk factors for future heart attacks. Such studies document associations between the occurrence of heart attacks and cigarette smoking, arterial hypertension, elevated serum cholesterol, Type A personality, etc. What still is lacking in the logic chain is the evidence that reducing the risk factors in a given individual will prevent the occurrence of coronary artery disease in that person. Dr. Ornish's research and that of others today is seeking the evidence for that missing link. Nevertheless, even with the data not yet all available, the prudent person will benefit his or her well-being, and very probably his or her heart as well, by adopting and adhering to the dietary and stress modification programs Dr. Ornish has presented in such a readable and attractive manner in this important book. I would go one step further in urging adoption of regular, moderate aerobic exercises—walking, cycling, jogging, swimming, etc.—together with the diet and stress modification that he recommends. We will be healthier as a nation and individually happier and more fulfilled to the extent that we follow his advice.

—ALEXANDER LEAF, M.D.

Chairman, Department of Preventive Medicine and Clinical Epidemiology, Harvard Medical School Chief, Medical Services, Massachusetts General Hospital (1966-1981)

Introduction

This book represents what I have learned from conducting two cardiovascular research studies at the Baylor College of Medicine, Houston, Texas, in 1977 and 1980.

My interest in this area of research began during my sophomore year of college in 1972, when I was trying to muddle my way through organic chemistry in hopes of going to medical school. I didn't enjoy organic chemistry, but it was one of the courses that was required by most medical schools.

On the first day of class, the professor told us, "You're not really here to learn chemistry. This is a weed-out course for the convenience of the medical school admissions committees. I will serve my role by weeding you out. If you do badly in this course, you are not likely to be accepted to any medical school."

College may be the "best years of your life," but times like this were definitely stressful. I was concerned that I was going to fail (and thereby lose my dream of becoming a physician), so I studied all the time. But the more I studied, the harder it became to remember the equations. I began to have difficulty sleeping, became anxious and depressed, and felt generally miserable. I began taking a friend's Valium.

"This is crazy," I thought. "Here I am, nineteen years old and starting to take tranquilizers—so I can learn to be a doctor." It was about that time when my older sister introduced me to her meditation teacher.

Perhaps meditation might help and it couldn't harm me, so I followed my curiosity to the first class. "Is that all there is to it?" I thought after the first session. But the teacher had an extraordinarily peaceful yet powerful presence, and I was convinced enough to continue practicing more or less regularly for six weeks.

There were no magic transformations, no cosmic visions or mystical experiences, but I noticed that gradually I was beginning to feel calmer and to think a little more clearly. While I never did learn to love organic chemistry, I was able to concentrate and to learn the material better. I no longer needed Valium.

I tend to be a pragmatic person. When someone teaches me something useful, I usually go back for more. "You'll find it easier to sit still and meditate if you cut back on the amount of animal products you eat," this teacher told me. At the time, this made no sense at all, but I thought, "Why not try it and see what happens?" Gradually, over the next several months, I modified my basic college diet of Kentucky Fried Chicken and McDonald's cheeseburgers to meals based at first on fish, and later primarily on fruits, vegetables, and whole grains.

Again, there were no dramatic experiences to report. My new way of eating did not improve my personality or my grades. But I did feel calmer yet more energetic.

In 1975, I began my first year of medical school at Baylor. One of the nicest aspects of this medical school was that the curriculum was very flexible. I chose a course of study that allowed me to take the basic science courses over two years instead of one, allowing me some free time to think and read outside the classroom.

During my first year at Baylor, I participated in a new branch of the American Medical Students Association (AMSA) for medical students who were interested in preventive medicine and health education. We exchanged ideas and reprints of interesting research articles via periodic newsletters and at AMSA's annual national convention.

Through these interactions, I began to read the work of investigators such as Drs. Herbert Benson and Bernard Lown (discussed later in this book) at the Harvard Medical School. I became excited by their findings, which indicated that meditation could be beneficial in treating high blood pressure (hypertension) and irregular heartbeats (arrhythmias).

The work of a British physician and scientist, Chandra Patel, M.D., was especially interesting. She studied a combination of stress management techniques based on yoga—meditation, breathing, and progressive deep relaxation—in treating some of

2

her hypertensive patients. Dr. Patel found that these stress management techniques could significantly reduce blood pressure and serum cholesterol independent of dietary changes.

At the Channing Laboratory (affiliated with Harvard Medical School and the Brigham and Women's Hospital), Drs. Frank Sacks, William Castelli, Edward H. Kass, and their colleagues studied a group of Americans who had been eating a primarily vegetarian diet for long periods of time. They found that blood pressure and serum cholesterol values were much lower in this group than in the general population. These levels of cholesterol and blood pressure were similar to populations of countries in which coronary heart disease is rare.

In summary, then, these studies indicated that stress management techniques, such as meditation, may reduce both blood pressure and serum cholesterol independent of changes in diet, and that a diet low in animal products may reduce both blood pressure and serum cholesterol independent of changes in stress.

(In other studies, Dr. Sacks and his associates more recently discovered that when this group of vegetarians was fed a diet high in animal products for several weeks [with the same amount of sodium as the vegetarian diet], the average blood pressure and serum cholesterol increased—independent of changes in stress. It was not surprising that a high-cholesterol diet caused the amount of cholesterol in the bloodstream to increase—but the changes in blood pressure were unexpected.)

In 1976, Drs. F. R. Ellis and T. Sanders in England reported that they treated four patients who had chest pain (angina) with a diet very low in animal products. At the end of five months, these patients experienced complete relief of chest pain and were able to engage in strenuous activities without difficulties. (A followup study five years later showed no return of these symptoms.)

The stress reduction techniques and the diet used in all of these studies were derived from yoga techniques that have been practiced in combination for centuries, so it made sense to study them together rather than one at a time. In 1977, I took a one-year leave of absence from Baylor and planned a small pilot study to measure the effects of a program that combined all of these components—stress management training and a diet low in animal products—in treating coronary heart disease, rather than just the risk factors for the disease, such as blood pressure and cholesterol levels.

Introduction

I discussed the project with several of the cardiologists at Baylor who were very generous with their time, resources, and constructive criticism. Dr. Antonio Gotto and others at Baylor agreed to support the study and donated most of the facilities for the evaluation testing that we performed.

In this pilot study, as described in Chapters 1–3, we documented numerous improvements in cardiovascular status in most of the patients—but why these changes occurred so rapidly was a mystery. At that time, these results could not be explained by the existing concepts of what caused coronary heart disease.

During the next three years (1978–1980), the understanding of coronary heart disease underwent a dramatic transformation. The important roles of coronary spasm and platelet clumping in causing coronary heart disease were documented (these are described in Chapter 4). Each of these mechanisms may be quickly activated by either emotional stress or dietary factors. While there was—and still is—controversy regarding how large a role each mechanism plays, both offered an explanation of how the improvements that we observed in our pilot study could have occurred so rapidly simply by reducing stress and changing diet.

Once these mechanisms became known, we were especially curious to know if stress management training and dietary changes could produce measurable improvements not just in how people felt or in risk factors such as cholesterol or blood pressure, but in the heart's function. Fortunately, recent advances in nuclear cardiology provided us with non-invasive tests that allowed us to monitor and assess the heart's function. Because of the favorable results from the pilot study, we planned a second study to see if such improvements could be documented.

We planned this study to overcome the limitations of the earlier one. With these new tests, we could now learn whether the patients were physiologically improving or if they only felt better. We included a larger number of patients and a randomized control group—that is, a comparable group of patients that we tested but who did not receive the program—in order to show that whatever changes we measured were due to the intervention and had not occurred because the patients would have improved anyway.

Part One of this book describes the results of our studies. Part Two is a step-by-step handbook that will show you how to implement the program.

The program consists of several parts, all of which interrelate.

For simplicity, however, it can be divided into two major components: stress management techniques and diet.

Stress Management Techniques. The unifying purpose of these seemingly different techniques is to enable you to gain progressively more awareness and control over your body and mind. Because it is easier to gain control over the body than the mind we begin with *stretching techniques.* These simple techniques can help to loosen up and remove some of the stress that we carry around as tension in our bodies. These are followed by a *progressive relaxation*, a sequential tensing and relaxation of all the muscle groups in the body, beginning at the feet and working up part by part to the head. This takes physical relaxation a step further and begins to remove stress from the mind as well.

Next there are a series of *breathing techniques.* Although it may seem unnecessary to teach anyone how to breathe, slow, deep, controlled breathing quiets the mind and body still further. By learning to control your breathing, you may gain more control over not only your body but also your mind.

By concentrating awareness on each inhalation and exhalation you begin to *meditate*, which simply means focusing the awareness on something—a word, the breathing, or a sound. As you gain progressively more control over the mind it can be directed away from negative or harmful thoughts. Also, it can be directed in a positive way—a double benefit. One way of doing this is known as *applied meditation* or *visualization*—focusing on a mental image of a desired state.

Diet. In our studies, the diet included no animal products except for small amounts of nonfat yogurt (which contains vitamin B_{12}, the only nutrient not available in a plant-based diet). Since cholesterol is found only in foods of animal origin, the diet was thus very low in cholesterol. Salt, sugar, alcohol, caffeine, and most processed foods were not included.

What the diet did include was fresh fruits and vegetables, whole grains, legumes (beans), and tubers (carrots, potatoes). It was high in complex carbohydrates, low in fat and cholesterol, and nutritionally complete. We paid particular attention to making the food attractive and appetizing.

My goal in writing this book is to explain what we did and what we found. It was not written to proselytize or convert, nor am I simply advising you to rigidly reject certain things that are considered "bad" and to accept only those that are considered "correct." For both the diet and the stress management techniques, there is a spectrum of possible participation and corresponding benefits. It is not all or nothing. I would encourage you to adapt whatever elements of the program seem useful for you at a rate of change that is comfortable. I hope that what we learned will help you to choose intelligently.

For example, foods from this program are classified in five groups (see pages 144–48). This is not a diet in the usual sense of the word—you are not "on" or "off" the diet. Based on our findings and the research of others, foods in Group 1 are considered to be the most healthful and those in Group 5 to be the least healthful, with Groups 2 through 4 intermediate. The more your diet is based on foods toward the Group 1 side of the spectrum, the more you are likely to benefit. (Of course, if you already have coronary heart disease you may wish to choose most of your foods from Group 1.) In our studies, the diet we served consisted only of foods from Groups 1 and 2.

The same principle applies to the stress management techniques. Just as with the diet, you may find that you like some techniques better than others. While the program works best as a whole, you should use only what you find appealing.

Coronary heart disease is largely a disease of excess—harmful reactions to chronic stress, and a diet based on excessive animal products. These chronically activate the web of mechanisms described in Chapter 4, which may reduce coronary blood flow and lead to the manifestations of coronary heart disease: chest pain (angina), heart attack, or sudden cardiac death.

The program is based on a simple concept: removing excess. Foods in Groups 1 and 2 of the diet are low in fat and virtually without cholesterol. With regard to stress, the program shows you how to react to stress in ways that are not harmful and how to remove physical and emotional tension when it occurs.

The choice is not between a productive, stressful, and interesting life that leads to coronary heart disease and sitting under a tree watching your life go by. This program will show you how you can increase your productivity and enjoyment—while reducing your risk of coronary heart disease.

Part One
THE PROGRAM

1. Overview

"The heart has reasons that reason knows not of . . .
do you love by reason?"

—BLAISE PASCAL, *Pensées* (1670)

"Men have become the tools of their tools."

—HENRY DAVID THOREAU (1817–1862)

This book describes a new program for treating and helping to prevent coronary heart disease. What distinguishes this program from others is that it has been tested in a controlled, scientific study and appears to produce improvements in the heart's function—without additional drugs or surgery.

The program is based on ancient stress management techniques and dietary changes. In an era of technological medicine, when the complex, expensive, and new are revered, it may seem odd that simple, inexpensive approaches that were first recorded thousands of years ago can be beneficial in treating coronary heart disease and relieving suffering. Yet they seem to be.

Along with my teachers and colleagues, we applied this program in treating patients who had advanced coronary heart disease. We measured the effects to see whether or not the patients improved. They did—and much more quickly than we expected.

We demonstrated for the first time in 1977, and more conclusively in 1980, that these patients experienced remarkable physical and emotional benefits in just a few weeks. Most participants reported a marked reduction in frequency and severity of angina pectoris (chest pain or discomfort due to heart disease); many became virtually pain-free for the first time in years. A follow-up survey revealed that these reductions in chest pain remained at this low level after six months. In many patients, backaches, headaches, and other chronic pains also decreased. Many reported an increased sense of general well-being and a renewed feeling of being in control of their lives. Many of those who wished to resume full-time work have been able to do so, even if they were severely disabled before beginning the program.

These changes were the most gratifying. However, the objective improvements were the most convincing and scientifically meaningful. We documented that most of our patients not only felt better, in many ways they *were* better.

We randomly divided a group of forty-six patients who had documented coronary heart disease into two groups: one group received the program for twenty-five days and the other did not. We tested both groups before and after the program, using advanced non-invasive instrumentation for evaluating cardiovascular function. Nuclear cardiology tests allowed us to indirectly visualize the heart beating and to calculate how well it was working.

Surprisingly, the heart's performance appears to have improved significantly in most of the patients who received the program. Also, we observed marked increases in exercise capability and significant reductions in blood pressure, weight, plasma cholesterol, and responsiveness to emotional stress. These changes occurred despite reductions in cardiac and antihypertensive medications in many of the participants. In contrast, the control group (which did not receive the program) did not improve.

The implications of these results are important. Coronary heart disease is not a small problem in this country. At least 40 million Americans are now suffering from heart and blood vessel diseases, including coronary heart disease, stroke, and hypertension. More than 600,000 Americans die each year of heart disease—almost one-half of all reported deaths, or almost as much as all other illnesses combined. Nearly one-quarter of fatal heart attack victims are below age sixty-five. Over 52 million workdays are lost each year to cardiovascular disease. Of course, these figures do not reflect the inestimable human suffering that cardiovascular disease brings to millions of people each year.

Of all the heart and blood vessel diseases, the vast majority (88 percent) are in the category known as coronary heart disease, in which the heart does not receive enough blood flow to maintain itself and becomes starved for oxygen. If the oxygen deprivation is for a brief time, then angina pectoris results: a sensation of tightness, choking, pressure, squeezing, or pain in the chest. If the reduction in blood flow is prolonged—more than a few minutes—then part of the heart may die: a heart attack. If a small part of the heart dies, then the dead portion becomes scar tissue and the person may continue to live. If it is a large area, or if it occurs in an important location of the heart, then the person may die.

What causes the reduction in blood flow to the heart? For the past fifty years or so, most physicians believed that it was almost entirely the result of a slow buildup of cholesterol and other deposits—like rust in a pipe—clogging the coronary arteries that supply the heart with blood. In recent years, however, it has been learned that the causes are not so simple. Other mechanisms besides fixed blockages in the coronary arteries can reduce blood flow to the heart. These include the roles of coronary artery spasm and platelet clumping, and they are described in detail in Chapter 4.

These mechanisms seem to be extremely sensitive to the effects of emotional stress and diet. Both the typical American diet and emotional stress, as well as cigarette smoking, may independently activate each of these mechanisms of coronary heart disease.

Coronary heart disease is usually treated with cardiac drugs and coronary bypass surgery. While these can benefit patients, alone they are insufficient in their approach.

For example, propranolol (Inderal), one of the most widely prescribed drugs, reduces the heart's need for oxygen by reducing its ability to pump blood. In doing so, it also may reduce the heart's ability to respond to exercise. In some patients, it can worsen lung disease and may cause heart failure, fatigue, depression, and impotence. It does nothing to increase the flow of blood and oxygen to the heart; it simply reduces the heart's consumption of oxygen by causing it to beat less vigorously.

In coronary bypass surgery, a vein is removed from the patient's leg and spliced to a coronary artery to provide a detour for blood around a blocked artery. Although coronary bypass surgery can thereby increase blood flow to the heart, it does so only by literally bypassing the problem and does nothing about the underlying causes of the disease.

The physical trauma and expense of coronary bypass surgery are considerable—and recent studies, including those by Dr. Richard S. Blacher of the Tufts–New England Medical Center, indicate that as many as one-third of heart surgery patients experience at least short-term postoperative emotional trauma. They often become delirious and have disturbing dreams and hallucinations, and a few may suffer enough anxiety and depression to contemplate suicide.

Many doctors are aware that emotional stress and a diet high in fat and cholesterol can lead to coronary heart disease via coronary artery spasm, platelet clumping, and other mechanisms. But most physicians believe, "There is not much you can do to reduce emotional stress, and you can't motivate patients to change their diet, at least not for long."

So, the majority of doctors prescribe drugs to reduce anxiety (Valium, Librium), drugs to lower cholesterol (clofibrate, cholestyramine), drugs to reduce platelet clumping (aspirin, Persantine), and newer drugs to reduce coronary artery spasm (nifedipine, verapamil). Rather than asking patients to decrease the intake of dietary cholesterol, a few surgeons even perform intestinal bypass surgery (cutting one end of the intestine where the cholesterol is absorbed and splicing it to a different part) to lower the amount of cholesterol in the blood.

Well, why not? What is wrong with drugs and surgery for treating coronary heart disease? Even if people could be motivated to reduce stress or change their diets, isn't it easier and quicker just to give them pills and operations?

There is nothing wrong with drugs and surgery per se. They can be lifesaving. When I am treating patients in the hospital, I prescribe drugs almost every day. And there are some patients with very severe or unstable coronary heart disease who may benefit from coronary artery bypass surgery. I am not suggesting that doctors should stop prescribing drugs nor that patients should stop taking them and avoid all surgical procedures.

The choice is not between technological medicine and the more ancient approaches described in this book. We need both—and the wisdom to know when each is appropriate. All of the elements in this program are compatible with the conventional medical and surgical therapies for treating coronary heart disease.

The debate regarding whether or not coronary bypass surgery prolongs life usually misses the point: compared to what? Studies which suggest that bypass surgery may prolong life compare these patients to those receiving only drugs, not those who have made major changes in their lifestyle and diet. The alternative to surgery is not just medical treatments; it includes the dietary changes and stress management techniques described in this book. The same is true for propranolol (Inderal), which has been shown in recent studies to substantially reduce the number of deaths following a heart attack. We need to stop thinking in either/or terms and use *everything* that is beneficial—including drugs and surgery when needed.

The point is simply this: by treating what appear to be the underlying causes of coronary heart disease using the program prescribed in this book, the progression of the disease may be modified and the need for drugs and surgery may be reduced. And for those who have bypass surgery, the program may help to keep the bypass grafts from clogging up. (Regression of fixed blockages in coronary arteries has been shown to occur in animals. A few preliminary studies suggest that this may be possible in humans, but much more evidence is needed.)

Problems arise because drugs and surgery are all too often given as substitutes for understanding and changing what I believe are the primary underlying causes of coronary heart disease: harmful responses to emotional stresses, a high-fat, high-cholesterol diet primarily based on animal products, and cigarette smoking.

Because these underlying causes are not often addressed, it is usually necessary to keep most heart patients on cardiac medications for the rest of their lives, often in ever-increasing dosages. Despite this, in most people the natural history of coronary heart disease (perhaps "unnatural history" would be more accurate) is to become progressively worse. The disease slowly and inexorably progresses in most patients. Neither cardiac drugs nor coronary bypass surgery do anything to slow this progression of the underlying disease. The following patient's story is typical of many:

"After my catheterization, the doctor told me that I had a sixty percent blockage of one of my coronary arteries. He said that the 'normal' buildup of plaque is about ten percent a year, so he wanted to do another catheterization in a year or two to take another look—and that in all probability I'd have to have a bypass. He didn't tell me anything about changing my diet or how to react to stress in a healthier way."

Most medical interventions occur after the fact, when a person

already has become sick. Medical technology is usually chan-
neled into treating, rather than preventing, coronary heart disease.
Unfortunately, in subtle and not so subtle ways, medical students
and residents often are taught that patients do not become
"interesting" until after they have developed a disease.

With only drugs and surgery, the best we can hope for is
symptomatic relief, a truce, a forestalling of further disease and
death. Following coronary bypass surgery, the blockages in the
coronary arteries tend to become progressively worse, and even
the bypass grafts can become clogged, often requiring additional
surgery. As the noted cardiologist Dr. Henry McIntosh wrote in
an article surveying the last ten years of bypass surgery, "Because
bypass surgery does not reverse the basic pathologic process of
atherosclerotic occlusive disease, it represents at best a new lease
on life which is temporary. The procedure is palliative rather
than curative or preventive." Dr. Denis Burkitt, an eminent
British surgeon, often ends his lectures by showing a cartoon of
a group of doctors feverishly moppng up a flooded floor (using
the most advanced techniques and equipment) rather than simply
turning off the faucet in the overflowing sink.

Mopping the floor can be quite expensive. Health care costs
have risen far out of proportion to the rate of inflation, from an
annual total of about $12 billion in 1950 to a stratospheric $200
billion in 1981, and there is no end in sight.

In 1980 alone, heart disease patients paid more than $50
billion in related medical costs. Coronary arteriography testing
costs the nation about $500 million annually. The price of each
coronary bypass operation is at least $15,000 to $20,000, and
from 1975 to 1980 more than 540,000 were performed. In 1980,
the annual cost of coronary bypass surgery in just the United
States was over *$2 billion*, and some analysts have predicted on
the basis of present trends that within twenty years the operation
could be a *$100 billion per year* industry.

Efforts to contain health care costs in this area have been
largely ineffective because they do not address the more fundamental problem: Is there a better way to treat coronary heart
disease? Health care delivery (perhaps "disease care delivery"
would be more accurate) soon will become the largest industry in
the country.

Our program takes a different approach. It does not "deliver"

14

coronary health care—it helps you to begin healing yourself. It is inexpensive, requires no special equipment or advanced technology, and is without trauma or dangerous side effects. In these respects, it is the opposite of many current medical practices. It is based on the premise that removing what seem to be the causes of coronary heart disease—turning off the faucet—is a better approach then just treating the disease.

Our bodies and minds are capable of reversing much of the damage we inflict on them if given a chance to do so—and more quickly than we had believed possible in the past. Unfortunately, we seldom give ourselves this chance. Three times a day (or more), when we eat, we continue to (literally) fuel the problem; likewise, stress seems to be a constant in our lives. This program can provide you with the chance to begin healing yourself.

Of course, a lifetime of abuse cannot be completely reversed overnight—but you will be surprised at how quickly you may notice improvements. If you do not yet have coronary heart disease, this program will likely reduce your risk of developing it. (Other types of heart disease—valvular disease, cardiomyopathy, or congenital defects—are unlikely to improve from this program.)

As with all research, our study has its limitations. We are not able to separate the relative contribution of each part of the program. Taken as a whole, it works very well, but it may be that some parts are more important than others. Since each person is a unique individual, it is likely that the contribution of each mechanism causing heart disease varies from person to person; therefore, some people may respond to different aspects of the program more than others. Also, our objective findings need to be reproduced by other investigators and on a larger scale before they can be considered definitive, but it will be years before this is completed. In the meantime, we all need to eat and to cope with stress.

There is a large body of related scientific research evidence that supports our conclusions. In fact, the evidence is so overwhelming that a leading researcher in this field, Jeremiah Stamler, M.D., wrote recently in *Circulation*, a cardiology journal, "Given the vast body of consistent information from many research methodologies on the relationship between lifestyle and atherosclerotic [coronary heart] disease, it is inappropriate to use the term *hypothesis* in speaking about this general area of knowledge. . . . A hypothesis is a conjecture. . . . [It is] a *theory*, a more or less verified or established fact or phenomenon."

For example, in 1982 Dr. I. Hjermann and his colleagues reported the results of a study of twelve hundred men forty to forty-nine years of age who were at high risk of developing coronary heart disease. After five years, they demonstrated that reducing cigarette smoking and the amount of animal products in the diet produced a 47 percent lower rate of heart attacks and sudden cardiac death than in a comparable group of men who served as controls.

If there is so much evidence, then why do most doctors still treat patients who have coronary heart disease primarily with drugs and surgery, and why is so little emphasis placed on lifestyle modification?

Dr. Alexander Leaf, Professor of Medicine and Preventive Medicine at Harvard Medical School, summarized it well when he stated: "Our profession, through a chain of events in the past thirty to forty years, has slipped into a posture of responding to human dis-ease with pills or surgery. These responses to patients' complaints seem to be emotionally satisfying and fiscally remunerative, so why change? There are many factors which understandably cause conservatism among physicians."

In a real sense, we have exchanged the power to manipulate the world through technology for the understanding of what it means to be *a part of* the world rather than *apart from* it. By developing a perspective that accumulates more and more information about less and less, we have gained a tremendous amount of power. What we have lost in the process *is* the process—the vision of the interdependence and balance of our world, and in particular, of our bodies and minds.

This is especially true in cardiology, where for the last two hundred years scientists and physicians have focused so intently on the heart itself that they tended to ignore the fact that it was connected to the brain. With our modern instruments we can scrutinize the coronary arteries in a living heart, we can examine pieces of the heart magnified a million times or more, and we can monitor the heart's electrophysiology, but we have no tools for viewing what goes on inside the mind, even though ultimately this may be far more important. Until just a few years ago, the investigation of the interaction between mind and body

16

was viewed as unscientific, "soft," or even metaphysical, not really worthy of scientific study since it cannot be measured and quantified.

But this limited perspective is changing. As Dr. Bernard Lown, a renowned cardiologist, wrote in an article on sudden cardiac death: "To date, research has been focused exclusively on the heart as the seat of deranged function. In fact, the focus should be shifted from the heart as target to the brain as trigger. . . . The therapeutic implications are profound."

Also, there is a human tendency—accentuated in industrialized societies like ours—not to value something unless it is new or expensive. After a while, that which is inexpensive and ancient tends to be forgotten (unless it is rediscovered and given a new name or new packaging).

Likewise, most medical students quickly absorb the mythology that it is more emotionally rewarding to do things *to* patients than to teach them what they can do to help themselves. Behind the white jacket and the reserved clinical façade, many of us physicians want to be the knight on the white horse who saves his patients from death and disease. Patients expect the doctor to *do something*. So there is a subtle but real bias against approaches that lessen the patient's dependence upon the doctor and his procedures. Also, powerful economic pressures can unwittingly bias physicians. After all, it is only human to be more enthusiastic about studying and implementing a procedure that generates $2 billion annually than one that costs very little.

Many physicians believe that they are truly helping their patients even though they are often unwittingly fostering a sense of dependence on themselves. Yet prolonged dependence often leads to weakness and can make patients feel that they are helpless victims of disease. Ironically, this weakness can foster disease in a vicious cycle.

Both doctors and patients tend to view pain as an enemy to be vanquished rather than as a message that something is wrong and needs to be corrected. According to legend, the ancient Romans killed any messengers who brought bad news. We have a tendency to respond to pain the same way—which is somewhat like clipping the wires to a ringing fire alarm rather than putting out the fire. Both patients and physicians have been conditioned to expect instant relief rather than to search for and address the underlying causes of the pain.

What makes technological medicine so appealing is that it often offers instant relief of pain. Nitroglycerin relieves most episodes of chest pain in just a few minutes. Most patients are pain-free following coronary bypass surgery. But because the underlying problems are not corrected, the coronary heart disease usually progresses and the pain tends to recur. Worse, this approach reinforces the erroneous belief that your health is something that a doctor or a pill can give you. (I have seen patients hold up their bottle of nitroglycerin and say, "My health is inside this little bottle.")

Lasting well-being does not usually come from pills, or from anything external. This program does not give you any new external things—because in the long run that is not what you need to be healthy. Rather, it simply helps you to identify and remove whatever is keeping you from being healthier.

Although we tend to view ourselves as fundamentally lacking and never quite having enough, coronary heart disease is in many respects an illness of excess—too much of the wrong foods, too many cigarettes, and too much anxiety and stress from viewing and reacting to the world in harmful ways. In this context, pain (whether physical or emotional) can be viewed as an aid in helping to identify whatever is contributing to the disease. The stress management techniques do not bring health; they simply aid in identifying and removing whatever is disturbing it, allowing us to experience an inner sense of well-being. Likewise, the diet does not provide any magical nutrients that will ward off heart disease, because coronary heart disease is not caused by nutritional deficiency. Instead, it simply removes those parts of the diet that contribute to heart disease, giving the body a chance to heal itself.

The program also appears to be beneficial in treating adult-onset (Type II) diabetes mellitus. The work of other investigators, as well as our much more limited experience, suggests that many Type II diabetics who require insulin may reduce or even eliminate (under a doctor's supervision, of course) the need for daily insulin injections, especially when patients lose weight. The pancreas can regulate the body's need for insulin much more closely than even new devices such as automatic insulin pumps.

This is important not just because daily injections of insulin are painful, time consuming, and expensive. More important, the ravages of diabetes (diabetic retinopathy, neuropathy, kidney disease, and peripheral vascular disease) may be less likely to occur in patients whose blood sugar is well controlled without the need for insulin. Likewise, there is some evidence to suggest that a diet based on foods in Groups 1 and 2 may reduce the risk of developing certain types of cancers, especially cancer of the breast, colon, prostate, and uterus. However, since our research was limited to studying the effects of the program in treating coronary heart disease, this book will be primarily limited to this area.

Good health is not boring. In this book, you will see that the choice is not between living an exciting, productive life and dying young from a heart attack versus leading a boring, unrewarding life in a "low-stress environment" and surviving to a ripe old age. But the misconception remains. Long ago, Mark Twain reportedly asked his physician, "Doc, if I give up wine, women and song, will I live longer?" The doctor replied, "No, but it will *seem* longer." (To which Twain replied, "In that case, I may give up singing. . . .")

But what you gain from this program is more than what you give up. Unlike many health programs, the goal is not to live longer or to lose weight—although this program may help you to do both. It is to enjoy life *now*, more free of pain and disease. The emphasis is not on what you have (or have not) done in the past, but what you can do for yourself in the present.

Responsibility is a word that has been much misused lately as a term of blame. As one patient remarked, "It was bad enough feeling sick—I did not want anyone telling me that I contributed to my illness."

But to feel responsible is not to feel blame or guilt—it is to feel more liberated and powerful. To the degree that we understand how we are responsible for our well-being—for better and for worse—then we are free to do something about it. Of course, this is not to say that we have responsibility and control over everything, but we do to a greater degree than we previously have thought possible. We have the power to change. This book shows you why—and how.

19

2. Subjective Improvements

George B. is a husky sixty-four-year-old man. When I first met him in July 1980, he had been suffering from angina—the chest pains due to coronary heart disease—for five years. George was a security guard, but during the previous two years he was unable to work because of his chest pain and fatigue.

"I'm not up to it. I want to work but I can't," he said during our initial interview. "I have chest pain every day, after any exertion: shaving, after a shower, walking, lifting, trying to cut the grass. I'm tired, can't get started . . . don't feel like doing anything . . . just huffing and puffing. At home I couldn't do anything. All I was doing was laying around the house. I didn't even go out in the yard. I would just sit and watch television all day. I didn't even have enough energy to get up and change the channels if I didn't like the show that was on."

George had been taking medication for his pain, but he had stopped for the four months before he entered the program. "The pills didn't seem to be doing any good. They would leave me even more tired. So I just gave them up."

For George, the inactivity caused by his physical pain was another source of stress. The frustration of being unable to work contributed to his angina, making him further incapacitated in a vicious cycle. "It kind of gets to you . . . because it's the same thing sitting around, day in and day out. You don't know what to do with yourself—you want to do something, you can't do it. There is always that obstacle . . . something holding you back.

You walk a block or two . . . you start to huff . . . to perspire . . . you just stop.''

"How does that make you feel?" I asked him.

"Tired, depressed, and disgusted. Sometimes I feel, 'I wish I'd fall asleep and in my sleep . . . just pass away.' ''

On Day 26 of our research program George described what he had experienced.

"They're very big changes for me. Now I have no pain whatsoever, even though I'm walking between two and three miles a day, with no weak feelings either. In fact, when I first came here, after the first two or three days I didn't have much pain. After about a week, I had none at all. And my mind is clearer—I seem to be waking up. I've snapped out of my depression ninety percent or more."

"Do you think you will be able to go back to work now?"

"Oh, yes, in fact it's not going to be long after I get out of here that I will be working."

"Do you still hope that you pass away in your sleep?"

"Oh, hell, no," he answered, a grin spreading across his face. "I feel too good to die."

After George returned home, he found a full-time job in security work and stayed on the program, doing well. "I've been feeling very good since coming back. No problems physically, no pain or anything, no huffing and puffing," he reported.

However, old habits are not easy to change. When the holiday season came, George began eating his former favorite foods—meatballs, hot dogs, hamburgers—and he stopped all of the stress management techniques he had learned. After a few days, his symptoms began to reappear. Over the next few weeks he began to experience increasing chest pain, a lack of energy, cramping in his legs due to insufficient blood flow, and symptoms of diabetes. Once again, he was unable to work.

I called him at that time to follow up on how he was doing, and he told me what was happening. I encouraged him to resume the program.

He did, and he experienced a rapid disappearance of virtually all his symptoms. He continues to do well and is working full-time.

*   *   *

His response to the program was not unusual. Frank M., a patient in our earlier study in 1978, had an experience similar to George's in several ways.

Frank M., a fifty-five-year-old commercial airline employee, suffered his first heart attack in 1965 and a second in 1970. Following his second heart attack, his cardiologist told him to work no more than four to six hours per day and restricted him to a desk job rather than the management training classes he had been teaching.

Frank had suffered severe angina since his second heart attack. Before beginning the program he said, "I have pain every day, sometimes twice a day. For the past eight years I've only been able to take tub baths, because by the time I'd be finished with a shower I'd be hurting so badly I'd have to take medication. I was practically living on nitroglycerin. Sometimes I'd have to take up to eight to get some relief.

"The pain is a very harsh tightening in the chest, with pains running down each arm. Right in the bend of both elbows it feels like someone's driving a nail or spike in there. It's very intense, so bad I would have been ready to scream if it would have helped."

Just before beginning the program, Frank had a flat tire on a Texas freeway. "The pain was so intense after changing the tire that I had to hold on to the car for support and almost pull myself back into the driver's seat to continue on to work. I broke out in a cold sweat."

Within a month after starting the program, he was able to change the alternator in his car without pain and without nitroglycerin. "By the end of the third week, I wouldn't have any pain at all unless I'd run, lift, or bend, but by the end of the fourth week I could do all of those things without pain. I couldn't run a hundred-yard dash, but I could walk along at a smart clip, which I hadn't been able to do for years."

The Thanksgiving and Christmas holidays came, and Frank also went off the program—and his pain returned. On January 4, 1978, he went to the hospital emergency room with what he thought was a heart attack. He was in the intensive care unit for two days. Fortunately, his pain turned out to be severe angina, not an actual heart attack. He was discharged on January 10 and went back on the program.

"I had no pains at all after three weeks back on the program," he said. "In the second week of February, I had another flat tire on a bigger car. I pulled over to a service station to have someone fix it, and they couldn't. So I crawled into the back, undid the new tire, took the jack out, carried it around, jacked the car up, changed the wheel, went back and put all the stuff back in the trunk, tightened it down, got out without a bit of pain, and went on home. No pain.

"Until you've had it, until you've gone through it, you don't know what it means to be free of that pain."

Three months later, Frank's cardiologist allowed him to return to full-time work for the first time in eight years.

George and Frank were not the only patients in our studies who felt better. By the end of both studies, most of the participants had improved, some more than others. Those who had the most severe disease and the largest degree of pain tended to improve the most—probably because they had the most room for improvement and the most motivation for continuing the program.

At the start of the second study, the participants reported an average of 10.1 episodes of chest pain per week. After two weeks, the frequency of angina had dropped to an average of only 1.6 pains per week, and two weeks after that to approximately 1 episode per week. One year later the angina frequency was still an average of about 1 episode per week.

Andrew G., a seventy-five-year-old man who participated in the first study, also experienced marked improvements. "I had my first heart attack in 1961. Since then, I've had three more. I've had angina [chest pain] since 1961—I would have severe pains once or twice a day, sometimes once or twice a week, but I can't remember a week going by without having some pain. I was running scared all the time.

"Since being on the program, I have had no chest pain. None. I've been testing myself. I've tried to do everything that would bring on a pain, and nothing's brought it on—lifting, walking rapidly, even into a jog trot, all these things that I'd been missing doing."

These were striking improvements. When I voiced my skepticism to Andrew, he replied, "If you were sitting here and I was listening to you, I'd call you either a blithering idiot or a liar. I would not believe you. But I am telling you the truth."

Because of his improvements, his cardiologist allowed him to return to his wheat farm for the first time in years. "My doctor has had me confined to under five hundred feet of altitude, but because I've improved so much in the program he's turned me loose so I can go back to Nebraska to the wheat farm harvest and into the mountains for a fishing trip or to hunt deer with my camera. I'm going to love getting back to that type of living."

Andrew stayed on the program during that month, and enjoyed his time in Nebraska without any problems. Unfortunately, a short time after he returned he felt so good that in spite of my strong urging to continue the program, he suddenly abandoned it.

"I'm cured," he said.

"No, you are not," I told him. "You are better, but to maintain these improvements, it is necessary to continue the program indefinitely."

"If any of the pains return—back, foot, or chest—then I'll resume it." Sadly, a few weeks after we spoke, he suddenly had a massive stroke, and he died shortly thereafter.

Was there cause and effect? Would he have had a stroke even if he had remained on the program? I do not know. However, new evidence indicates that some of the mechanisms which may cause coronary heart disease and strokes, including the role of platelet clumping, are very sensitive to short-term changes in diet and in emotional stress. These are discussed in detail in Chapter 4.

The program we followed during our study was intensive. We wanted to show the greatest effects in the shortest possible time. Therefore, we served foods from Groups 1 and 2 only. Stress management techniques were taught and practiced five hours a day. You probably will not have nearly so much time to practice these techniques as the patients had during our studies—but even if you can practice them for only a few minutes each day, you will benefit.

Here is the schedule we followed during our studies:

7:00– 7:45 A.M.   Stretching and breathing techniques
8:00– 8:45 A.M.   Breakfast

9:00–10:00 A.M.	Nutrition education (lecture)
10:30–11:00 A.M.	The roles of stress and diet in coronary heart disease (lecture)
11:00–11:30 A.M.	Breathing, meditation, and visualization
12:00– 1:00 P.M.	Lunch
1:00– 4:00 P.M.	Free time
4:00– 5:30 P.M.	Stretching, breathing, and progressive deep relaxation
6:00– 7:00 P.M.	Dinner
7:30– 9:00 P.M.	Group discussion, guest lectures, or entertainment

Nearly all of the patients felt that the program as a whole contributed to their improvements, but for some individuals certain aspects were more important than others. For some, it was the diet.

Fifty-seven-year-old Don S., an antiques dealer, entered the program weighing 287 pounds, with angina so severe that he had been taking an average of thirty to forty nitroglycerin tablets a week. By the end of the study his chest pain was so significantly reduced that he needed only three nitroglycerin tablets during the last seven days. He lost thirty pounds and was able to stop taking the ten units of insulin that he had been injecting each morning for years. "I have much more energy—I'm even looking at the young ladies again."

Don knew that the diet was an important part of the program for him. "The old way of cleaning up buffet tables is out—and I don't mean as a busboy, but as a champion of all eaters. I was the world's greatest gourmet. The only exercise I ever did was to pick up a fork. Food was my heroin.

"But those pains really frightened me. I realized that if I didn't change, I would probably die within a few years, or even worse—end up with a stroke and become incapacitated. Just keeping a person alive is not enough, though. You should enjoy life; you should have vigor and vitality even to old age. I chose to be as healthy as possible. The diet hasn't eliminated my enjoyment of food."

Six months after the study ended, Don had lost almost one hundred pounds "without effort." He has had almost no chest pain, and with his doctor's permission he's been able to stop many of his medications.

For other participants the stress reduction exercises were more important. When sixty-two-year-old Ellen W. began the program she told us, "In the last two months I've been having angina every day, usually so often that it seemed constant."

Ellen's pain was brought on by physical activity, but its primary cause was emotional stress. "I'm nervous at the office, especially when there are a lot of things going on. I get all uptight and I get this tightness in my chest, a pressure, as if something's really squeezing it.

"Before my heart disease was diagnosed, I used to think the pains were just nerves, but the more I tried to control them, the worse they got. I have not handled stress well at all since I was very young, and as the years have gone by, I have handled it less and less well. It has taken a tremendous toll on my body. I was aware of it, but I didn't think there was anything I could do other than just to stiffen my back and get over it. For a few years I felt like I didn't really particularly want to live on because of my emotional distress.

"Before the program, if I felt that pressure in my chest I would have just pushed on, ignored it, gone on with what I was doing until it became so unbearable I had to stop. Now, I have the tools to react differently. Whenever I feel the pressure beginning I ask myself, 'What am I doing? How am I reacting to stress in a way that's causing me to hurt?' Then, I go into another room and do the deep relaxation exercises, meditate—and the pain usually goes away."

Like Ellen, some of the other people who adopted the program found that in many ways it changed their ways of responding to the world. Now, they were able to cope with stressful situations in a healthier, more productive way.

Even more important, they found that their well-being and equilibrium were less easily disturbed. Events simply did not upset them the way they once had. Frank M. was typical of many of the patients when he said, "I used to have a very short temper and a very short fuse, and I'd go off any minute. I find now that I don't have that problem as much as I did. Of course, things still bother me sometimes, but when they do I just turn them off and go about my business."

Andrew G. came home one day to find that his house had flooded. "If this had been before the program and I'd found my home flooded with an inch of water on the floor, I doubt very much if I'd even have tried nitroglycerin—I would have immediately gone to Demerol because I'd have been hurting so bad. And here, I didn't take anything—not a thing."

"What did you do?"

"Just mopped up the floor. The next morning I went back to my home and found more water from the rain during the night, so I mopped it up, too."

Anne B., a seventy-year-old woman who took part in our first study, told me three years later, "You know, my whole attitude has changed. I used to get angry a lot, even though I never showed it. Now, nobody makes me mad. I have other things to think about."

"How can people develop that attitude?"

"If they would just look around them, and realize all they have—and what they could lose. So many little things are so unimportant."

Many of the participants in our studies came expecting the staff or the program to make them well. But we could take little credit for their improvements. We were there only as facilitators: to provide them with information and to help them understand how they could begin to help themselves. The program detailed in this book can help you to do the same.

3. Objective Improvements

"There is only one quality worse than hardness of heart
and that is softness of head."

—THEODORE ROOSEVELT

As impressed as we were by these subjective changes, from a scientific point of view we were more interested in the objective measurements. Medical history is filled with techniques that made people feel better yet did not alter the underlying disease process.

As mentioned earlier, we conducted a pilot study of our program in 1977, with ten patients. We measured frequency of chest pain, blood pressure, exercise tolerance, and plasma cholesterol and triglyceride levels. The patients showed improvement in all of these objective measurements. We were excited by these changes, but knew that they could have been caused by a number of factors. We still did not know whether or not the heart itself was improving. In a few patients, we performed a test (described later) that gave some evidence that blood flow to the heart was improving.

In our second study, therefore, we performed a new test on all the participants that provided specific information about the heart's function: the amount of blood the heart pumps with each beat and how uniformly it contracts. Both of these are indicators of how much blood flow the heart is receiving.

In order to understand these tests, let's review how the heart works.

The heart is a pump. It is also a muscle. Like all muscles, it requires oxygen for fuel. To supply its own needs, the heart first pumps blood and oxygen to itself through the coronary arteries. The heart also pumps blood to the other parts of the body in order to supply the various tissues and organs with oxygen and other nutrients.

When a person begins to exercise, the body begins to use oxygen at a much faster rate—just as a car requires more gasoline to go faster. To meet the body's increased demand, the heart pumps blood more rapidly and forcefully. As a result, the oxygen requirements of the heart also increase dramatically.

In a healthy person this is not a problem: the heart receives enough blood through its coronary arteries to supply its increased demand for oxygen. When a person with coronary heart disease begins to exercise, however, his partially clogged coronary arteries are already supplying as much blood to the heart as they can. They are unable to admit enough extra blood to keep pace with the stepped-up demand, so the heart pumps less effectively.

Even a person who has moderately severe coronary heart disease may be getting enough blood flow to his heart when he is at rest—although just barely. Therefore, most tests which measure blood flow to the heart and its ability to pump blood can appear normal while a person is resting, even if he has coronary heart disease. When he begins to exercise, however, the heart pumps less effectively. As described above, the heart is unable to keep pace with the increased demand. So, most tests are more accurate when performed during exercise, since this makes the underlying coronary heart disease more apparent.

This is why electrocardiograms (EKGs) are taken not only at rest but also while running on a treadmill. However, these tests have a rather large margin of error. Some people with heart disease are not detected, and some people who do not have disease have false positive tests.

Until recently, the only way to directly measure the extent and severity of coronary heart disease in a patient was by cardiac catheterization. In this test, a small tube is threaded through an artery in the arm or leg until it reaches the heart. Dye is then injected through the tube into the coronary arteries, and an X-ray movie is made which shows if there are any blockages, and if so, their extent and location.

The test is accurate, but it is also very invasive and somewhat dangerous to the patient—at least one out of every thousand patients dies during this test even in the most experienced hands, and the incidence of major complications is much higher. In addition, the test usually only measures fixed blockages, rarely the extent of disease contributed by other factors such as coronary artery spasm and platelet clumping (described in the next chapter). Also, this test is not usually performed during exercise.

Most of the participants in our study were tested in this manner by their cardiologists for diagnostic rather than research purposes. We did not repeat this test after the program because of the complications associated with it—even though we were very curious to know if improvements were occurring in the hearts of the participants.

Fortunately, in recent years new non-invasive tests have been developed that allowed us to observe a patient's heart and calculate how well it was working at rest and during exercise. Two of the best are known as "thallium testing" and "gated blood pool studies."

A thallium test enables a doctor to see areas of the heart that are not getting enough blood flow. While running on a treadmill, the patient's vein is injected with an extremely small but measurable amount of thallium (an isotope) at the point of maximum exercise, when the oxygen demands of the heart are greatest. The thallium is carried in the bloodstream to the heart. Any areas of the heart that are not receiving sufficient blood flow will receive less thallium as well.

This can be directly viewed on a special video screen, where the changes in blood flow to the different parts of the heart are seen as variations in brightness. The lighter the area, the greater the blood flow; darker areas correspond to reduced blood flow.

Because of the expense, we performed thallium testing on only a few of the patients in the 1977 pilot study. We were surprised to find that after just one month some of these patients demonstrated an increase in blood flow to the heart during peak exercise.

The photographs on the opposite page show the results of this test in one of these patients. Figure 1 is a picture of his heart and lungs before he began the program. Arrow A points to an important area (the septum) that is not receiving much blood flow, so it is quite dark.

Figure 2 is a picture of the same heart and lungs, after the patient had followed the program for one month, but made no changes in medication. You can see how much more blood this area is

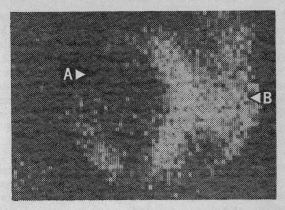

Figure 1

receiving now (Arrow A), even though the patient was exercising more during this test than he was during the first test. Although the heart was still not normal, the improvement was considerable.

Thallium testing also provides another measure of the extent of coronary heart disease. In patients who have very severe coronary heart disease, the heart's function deteriorates so much during exercise (because of inadequate blood flow through the

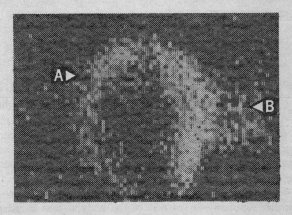

Figure 2

coronary arteries) that it cannot adequately pump blood through the lungs. This is seen in Figure 1: Arrow B points to the lungs, which appear too bright. The blood is "backed up" into the lungs because the heart is pumping so poorly. In Figure 2, one month later, the lungs appear more normal because the heart is pumping more effectively, so less blood is pooled in the lungs.

While these results were very interesting, they still were not sufficient proof. We tested only a small number of patients in this way and could not be certain that the improvements were due to the program. It is possible, though not very likely, that the patients may have gotten better anyway.

The best way to determine whether or not a treatment is effective is by what is called the scientific method of investigation. While it is not possible to measure everything, this approach provides a discipline for evaluating new treatments by decreasing the number of alternative explanations and by reducing the chance that possible experimenter bias (prejudice) might influence the results.

A randomized, controlled study is a rigorous way of doing this. In this design, volunteers are randomly divided into two groups: one receives the program (the experimental group), and the other (the control group) does not. Both groups are tested before and after the program. Since the patients are randomly assigned, the two groups should be comparable in most respects except that one group receives the program and the other does not. Therefore, it can safely be assumed that any differences between test results in the two groups are most likely due to the program and not to other factors. Also, the more patients that are included in each group, the more likely it is that they represent the general population of people who have coronary heart disease, and thus the more evidence there is for generalizing the findings.

As discussed in the Introduction, we repeated our research in 1980 with a larger number of patients and a randomized control group. All of the participants were tested with what are called "gated blood pool studies," a more quantitative measurement of the heart's function than thallium testing.

With each beat, the heart pumps blood from its main chamber— the left ventricle—to the rest of the body. Gated blood pool studies measure the percentage of blood that the heart ejects

32

(pumps) from the ventricle with each beat. This percentage is called the "ejection fraction."

In a healthy person at rest, the heart pumps at least half of the blood from its main chamber with each beat. (The other half remains in the heart.) That is, the ejection fraction is at least 50 percent. As he begins to exercise, the heart will pump a greater percentage of blood with each beat in order to supply more blood to the body—at least 5 percent more in most healthy people. In other words, in a healthy person the ejection fraction will rise at least 5 percent during exercise when compared to the ejection fraction at rest.

However, in a person with coronary heart disease, the ability of the heart to pump blood deteriorates during exercise. The diseased heart simply cannot keep pace with the increased demands of exercise. Thus, the ejection fraction does not rise at least 5 percent during peak exercise. If the heart disease is severe, it may even fall while exercising. So, the ejection fraction response to exercise provides a sensitive and specific means of measuring the presence and severity of coronary heart disease.

Before beginning our program, the patients' gated studies showed a slight fall in average ejection fraction during exercise. This is what we expected, since previous tests (cardiac catheterization, electrocardiography, and so forth) documented that they had coronary heart disease.

After twenty-five days of the program, we were delighted to find that the ejection fraction no longer fell with exercise—it rose an average of 5.8 percent. In contrast, the control group (which did not receive the program) did not improve. This was evidence that the heart's function had probably improved due to the program. (These changes in ejection fraction were similar to a comparable group of patients who were studied in the same laboratory before and two weeks after coronary artery bypass surgery.) A more detailed description of our findings is found in the Appendix.

Besides calculating the ejection fraction, gated studies provide a second way of evaluating the extent of coronary heart disease: a moving picture of the heart as it contracts. In a gated study, a computer-generated movie is made of the beating heart at rest and during exercise. If any areas of the heart are not contracting uniformly, these can be directly viewed and recorded.

In a healthy person, the heart will contract uniformly during each beat. However, in a person who has coronary heart disease, the parts of the heart that are not receiving enough blood flow will not contract properly during each heartbeat. These parts will lag behind the rest of the heart's wall as it contracts. If the disease is very severe, these sections of the heart may even bulge outward rather than contracting inward during each beat.

As described earlier, when a person with coronary heart disease begins to exercise, his heart cannot keep pace with the increasing demands on it. As a result, new areas of abnormal contraction appear in the heart during exercise that are not present at rest. The presence of these new areas of abnormal contraction in the heart that appear during exercise is a sensitive measurement of the presence and severity of coronary heart disease.

As we expected, most of the patients in our study displayed new abnormal areas in the heart during exercise when we studied them before they began the program. After twenty-five days of the program, there was a significant improvement in these abnormal areas when compared with the group that did not receive the program—more evidence that the program caused improvements in the heart's function.

These improvements occurred even though most of the patients exercised 44 percent longer and performed 55 percent more work after twenty-five days of the program, and even though they had reduced or even discontinued much of their cardiac and high blood pressure medications. (We had not planned to reduce these medications during the study, but it became necessary to do so when many of the patients began to show side effects and excessively low blood pressure, even though the dose and frequency of their medicines were not increased. Patients simply did not seem to need as much medication after being on the program.)

We also measured other improvements. Blood pressure was significantly reduced, not only at rest, but also in response to a variety of emotionally stressful stimuli. Also, the amount of cholesterol in the blood was significantly lowered, from an average of 229 to 182 mg percent. Many studies have shown that, in general, the higher a person's blood pressure, and the higher his serum cholesterol, the greater is his risk of developing coronary heart disease, stroke, or a heart attack. The reverse is also true. Therefore, it is reasonable to assume that those patients who maintain these lower levels of blood pressure and cholesterol may be increasing their life expectancy, all other factors being equal.

We also measured a variety of psychological improvements. Drs. Meyer Friedman and Ray Rosenman have described what they termed "Type A behavior," characterized by competitiveness, hostility, time urgency, and other characteristics. They have found that patients with Type A behavior are at a higher risk for developing coronary heart disease. In our study, we found that patients' behavior became less Type A, even though we had not tried to change their behavior in this way. The reasons for these changes are explored further in the next chapter. In addition, tests of psychological well-being demonstrated significant improvements.

Studies by Dr. Ralph Paffenbarger, Dr. Dieter Kramsch, and others suggest that moderate aerobic exercise may help to prevent coronary heart disease in people who do not yet have it. Aerobic exercise—especially walking—can be a useful addition to this program, but it is not a substitute for changing diet and harmful reactions to stress. Unless these also are modified, intensive aerobic exercise can be potentially risky for people with coronary heart disease.

Regular, moderate physical activity is a good idea for most people. In some people with coronary heart disease, however, exercise is associated with a small but definite increased risk of heart attacks, arrhythmias, and sudden death. While the risks for those without heart disease are minimal, many people are not aware that they have coronary heart disease until it is too late. Therefore, exercise programs for people over forty should be supervised by physicians who are trained to monitor for these potentially lethal complications.

So, I have not included aerobic exercise as a formal part of this book. The first principle of medicine is "First do no harm." Since I cannot be certain that everyone with coronary heart disease who reads this book will be adequately supervised, I would rather forgo the potential benefits of vigorous aerobic exercise than risk possible lethal complications resulting from my recommendations here. Everything which I have included in the program is without significant risk. For most people, though, walking can be safely recommended, and for those under forty without known coronary heart disease, more vigorous aerobic exercise is advisable.

The next chapter describes in detail how emotional stress and the typical American diet are causes of coronary heart disease and why stress management training and dietary changes can produce the improvements we have seen.

4. What Is Coronary Heart Disease and How Do Stress and Diet Help to Cause It?

"A merry heart doeth good like a medicine: but a broken spirit drieth the bones."

—KING SOLOMON, Proverbs 17:22

"Every affection of the mind that is attended with pain or pleasure, hope or fear, is the cause of an agitation whose influence extends to the heart."

—WILLIAM HARVEY, De Motu Cordis (1628)

This chapter describes how stress and the typical American diet are causes of coronary heart disease. The causes of coronary heart disease are explored here in greater detail, including the newly understood roles of coronary artery spasm and platelet clumping.

As discussed in the previous chapter, your heart is a muscle. Oxygen is its main fuel, just as gasoline is the fuel that powers your car. Because your heart is always beating, it requires a continual supply of fuel (oxygen). Since oxygen is carried in the bloodstream, the heart needs a continual supply of blood, which it pumps to itself through blood vessels called coronary arteries.

What is coronary heart disease? Simply this: the heart does not receive enough blood flow to maintain itself. It becomes starved for the oxygen that is carried in the blood.

If the oxygen deprivation is for a brief time, then angina pectoris results—in a poetic sense, the heart is cryi. .g out in pain. This is usually described as a discomfort, heaviness, pressure, smothering, tightness, choking, or squeezing in the chest. The heart has been injured, but at this point the damage is reversible. This discomfort usually occurs during physical or emotional stress and is relieved by rest.

However, if the blood flow to part of the heart is reduced for more than a few minutes, then that area of the heart which is deprived of blood may die. This is called a myocardial infarction, commonly known as a heart attack. As stated earlier, if only a small part of the heart dies, then the dead portion becomes scar tissue and the person may live. If a large area of the heart is affected, or if it occurs in an important location, then a more serious outcome may result, including death.

What causes the reduction in blood flow to the heart?

Until recently, most of what physicians knew about coronary heart disease was learned only at the autopsy table. Here, the coronary vessels could be dissected and the blockages examined.

Because these people had died, only the structural changes in their coronary arteries could be studied. The minute-to-minute fluctuations in coronary blood flow that occur in a living heart— and the causes for these changes—could not be observed. Because of this, for the past fifty years or so most physicians believed that reduced blood flow to the heart was caused by only one mechanism: clogged coronary arteries.

Cholesterol and other substances in the blood can become deposited on the inner walls of the coronary arteries—like the buildup of rust in a pipe. These deposits are called plaque.

Over a period of years, these deposits can slowly increase. Eventually, the diameters of the coronary arteries become narrowed until the vessels no longer can carry enough blood to meet the requirements of the beating heart.

Physicians and scientists have long suspected that this buildup of plaque may not be the only mechanism that causes a reduction in blood flow to the heart. There were many clues. For example, it has been known for years that the degree of blockage in the coronary arteries does not correlate very well with the degree of symptoms that a person experiences. Some people with severely blocked coronary arteries do not have much chest pain, whereas others with only minor obstructions may have angina that is severe and frequent. Pathologists were especially puzzled by some people who had chest pain or died from heart attacks yet had no blockages at all in their coronary arteries.

During the past five years, however, diagnostic equipment has been developed that makes it possible to examine the living heart. It has now been shown that other mechanisms besides fixed blockages can reduce the blood flow to the heart. Recently, many of these mechanisms have been well documented. The most important of these involve (1) *coronary artery spasm*, and (2) *platelet clumping*. These, in turn, may be activated by other mechanisms.

Several investigators have found that emotional stress and a diet high in animal products may each cause fixed blockage formation, coronary artery spasm, and platelet clumping to occur. All of these mechanisms that cause coronary heart disease are interdependent—that is, they affect one another in many different ways. So, it is a mistake to view coronary heart disease as the result of one cause—rather, it appears to be the result of a *web* of interactions.

There are hundreds of research studies that document how emotional stress and diet may activate these mechanisms. However, most scientists have concentrated on studying only one or two of these mechanisms. These studies are enormously helpful, but they describe only fragments of the entire process. It is important to have a complete picture showing how all of these mechanisms interrelate.

What is coronary artery spasm? Your coronary arteries—like the arteries throughout your body—are not just pipes or conduits. The walls are lined with smooth muscle that can go into spasm, shutting down the flow of blood. The more fixed blockage there is in a coronary artery, the less spasm is required to completely close it off. Also, coronary artery spasm may cause part of the fixed blockage to rupture, causing blood to flow rapidly within the blockage (plaque hemorrhage). This can cause the blockage to rapidly expand, closing off the coronary artery.

What is platelet clumping? Blood platelets are the body's first defense against bleeding—they are the cellular components of the blood that help it to clot. When you cut yourself, platelets clump (aggregate) together inside the blood vessel that is bleeding, helping to stop the flow of blood. This also may occur inside the coronary arteries—a thrombosis—which can reduce or stop the flow of blood to the heart.

The discovery of these mechanisms a few years ago revolutionized the understanding of coronary heart disease. For the previous fifty years, this disease had been viewed as a static process, with deposits slowly building up over a long period of time

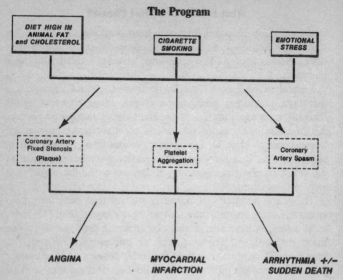

Figure 3. An overview of the main causes of coronary heart disease.

without much hope for improvement. Now it is seen as a *dynamic* process—for better and for worse.

Changes in coronary spasm and platelet function can increase or decrease the blood flow to the heart very rapidly—sometimes in a matter of seconds. As we will see, these mechanisms help to explain why, for example, chest pain or a heart attack often occurs during times of emotional stress or immediately following a large, high-fat, high-cholesterol meal. Although the role of fixed blockages is very important, it is not the only mechanism that causes angina and heart attacks.

In planning our study, we reasoned that reducing emotional stress and changing diet may improve cardiovascular function in patients with severe coronary heart disease via these mechanisms, and that this might occur very quickly. We would not have to wait for years to document these changes.

This appears to have happened. While we did not study the mechanisms for the cardiovascular improvements that we observed, there is considerable evidence from other investigators to indicate that these rapid changes may have been due to reductions in coronary spasm and platelet clumping. (The precise contribution of these mechanisms in causing angina and heart attacks is currently the subject of intense debate among research scientists.)

Our program addresses all of the known mechanisms that cause coronary heart disease and sudden death. While some benefit can be gained by addressing only a few of these, you can see why a combined approach makes more sense.

First, let's examine the evidence that emotional stress can cause a reduction in blood flow to your heart via these mechanisms.

For perhaps millions of years, our bodies have evolved to respond to emotionally stressful situations in ways that can help us to survive. Stress elicits what is known as the "fight-or-flight" response. This was first described by Dr. Walter B. Cannon, a professor of physiology at the Harvard Medical School at the beginning of this century.

The fight-or-flight response is a series of physiological changes that occur in our bodies to prepare us to respond to stressful or

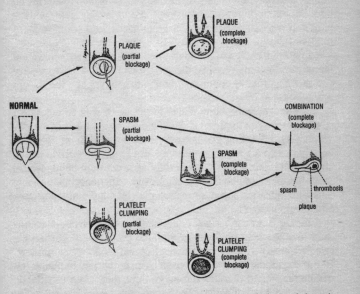

Figure 4. Causes of reduced blood flow to the heart: cholesterol deposits (plaque), coronary artery spasm, and platelet clumping. These may act independently or in combination.

dangerous situations. These changes include increases in heart rate, blood pressure, rate of breathing, muscular tension, and general metabolic rate. Coronary artery spasm and increased platelet clumping also can result from the fight-or-flight reaction.

As mentioned, some of these changes have survival value. For example, when our ancestors were being chased by tigers or were about to go into battle, it was very beneficial for arteries in their arms or legs to be more likely to go into spasm and for their platelets to be predisposed to clump together. If a person were wounded, arterial spasm and platelet clumping would help to stop the bleeding more quickly. Increased muscular tension helped to fortify the body's "muscular armor," offering more protection during a fight. It was useful for the heart to beat faster and for the metabolism to speed up because the body needed more oxygen and nutrients at these times. Of course, not all of these changes have survival value—and it is especially difficult to see the evolutionary advantage of having one's *coronary* arteries go into spasm during times of stress. Perhaps this represents a relatively recent response to the chronic stresses and diet of modern times.

Today, our bodies go through these changes whenever we are faced with genuine physical danger. However, twentieth-century stresses are usually emotional rather than physical—we do not often face real physical danger.

Unfortunately, the body reacts in the same way to emotional stresses as it does to physical ones. Now that the tigers are gone, we face different kinds of stresses. Whether we are angry at the boss, anxious about an impending deadline, or worried about unpaid bills, our bodies react exactly as if we were being chased by a tiger or were about to do battle—we experience increases in muscular tension, blood pressure, platelet clumping, coronary artery spasm, and so on.

Running from danger and doing battle are the physical actions for which the fight-or-flight reaction has prepared us. Our ancestors presumably responded by doing just that—fighting or running. But in the modern world, it is usually inappropriate to punch our competitors or to literally run away from them. We usually do not take this kind of action even though our bodies are geared to do so. Thanks to our imposed social and behavioral restraints, fight-or-flight has often become grin-and-bear-it.

Also, the stresses faced by our ancestors may have been more intense, but they probably were not as chronic. Being chased by a tiger may be more stressful than trying to compete in the business world—but it probably did not happen very often. Likewise, battles would be fought, but then they would be over.

Now, the battle never seems over—or one battle is soon replaced by another one. As a result, our fight-or-flight mechanisms are almost continually activated. Since we usually cannot take the appropriate physical actions, our bodies tend to be in a constant state of alarm.

Because these mechanisms are *chronically* activated, they become self-destructive, especially to the cardiovascular system. Rather than help us to survive danger, the fight-or-flight response may create it for us by causing coronary artery spasm and platelet clumping to occur. These mechanisms serve a useful and necessary function—they become harmful only because they are activated inappropriately. In this respect, the body is designed properly—we are simply abusing it.

How does stress cause coronary artery spasm to occur?

The nervous system is divided into two parts: the skeletal, or *voluntary* nervous system, and the *autonomic*, or so-called involuntary nervous system. When you want to move your arms or legs, your brain sends a message to them via the voluntary nervous system. The autonomic nervous system controls "automatic" functions of your body such as your heartbeat, breathing, and so on. (As described more fully in the discussion of meditation in Part Two, you can learn to control some aspects of your autonomic nervous system.)

The autonomic nervous system, in turn, is divided into two components: the *sympathetic* and *parasympathetic* nervous systems. These two systems tend to counterbalance each other. For example, stimulating your sympathetic nervous system causes your heart rate to increase and your arteries to constrict, while the parasympathetic nervous system causes your heart rate to decrease and your arteries to dilate. During times of stress, part of your brain (the hypothalamus) activates the fight-or-flight response by stimulating your sympathetic nervous system more than your parasympathetic nervous system.

How does the sympathetic nervous system work? These changes

in heart rate and arterial diameter are controlled by switches, or *receptors*, that are located on your heart and in your arteries. There are two types of these switches, called *alpha* and *beta* adrenergic receptors. ("Adrenergic" means they are activated by adrenaline [epinephrine], one of the stress hormones.) When the alpha receptors are stimulated, your arteries constrict; when the beta receptors are stimulated, your arteries dilate.

Norepinephrine, a stress hormone, turns on the alpha receptors—that is, it makes your arteries constrict, including the coronary arteries.

Norepinephrine is found in two different places:

1. Small packets of it are manufactured and stored in nerve endings of your sympathetic nervous system. These nerve endings are located next to the alpha receptors. During times of stress, your sympathetic nervous system is stimulated. This causes your nerve endings to release packets of norepinephrine, which bind to your alpha receptors and turn them on. This causes your arteries to constrict and your heart rate to increase.

2. Norepinephrine is also manufactured and stored in larger quantities by your adrenal glands (located next to your kidneys). During times of stress, your adrenal glands release norepinephrine and a related hormone, epinephrine (adrenaline), into your bloodstream. These hormones circulate and turn on alpha receptors throughout your body. This causes your arteries to constrict.

In 1973, Dr. Jacob Haft and his colleagues found that stress caused platelets to clump in the coronary arteries. How does stress cause this to occur?

Besides causing coronary artery spasm, norepinephrine and epinephrine are powerful stimulators of platelet clumping. Also, once the platelets begin to stick together, the platelets release a substance called *thromboxane* A_2. This is the most powerful substance in your body for causing platelet clumping to occur. Therefore, once platelets have begun to clump, more platelets can be stimulated to stick together in a self-perpetuating cycle.

When platelets clump together, they can lodge in the coronary arteries, obstructing blood flow to the heart (coronary thrombosis) or in the carotid arteries to the brain (stroke). When the arteries are already narrowed by fixed blockages, then this is more likely to occur.

Also, thromboxane A_2 has another important effect: it is the most powerful substance in the body that causes coronary artery spasm to occur. In this respect, it is even stronger than norepinephrine.

Any one of these mechanisms—platelet clumping, coronary artery spasm, and fixed blockages—may be sufficient to completely obstruct the flow of blood to the heart. The relative contribution of each mechanism seems to vary from individual to individual.

How does diet cause coronary artery spasm and platelet clumping to occur?

People with high levels of cholesterol have been shown to have platelets that are "stickier"—that is, their platelets clump together more readily than in patients with lower levels of cholesterol in their blood. A diet high in saturated fats can lead to increased platelet clumping. Even a single high-fat meal may cause acutely enhanced platelet clumping.

A diet that is high in fat and cholesterol—that is, the typical American diet—causes platelets to release increased amounts of thromboxane A_2. As we have seen, thromboxane can stimulate both coronary artery spasm and platelet clumping to occur.

Also, a high-fat diet results in elevated blood levels of *free fatty acids*, which are the building blocks of fat. The opposite is true with diets that are low in animal products (such as the foods in Groups 1 and 2 of the program).

Excessive free fatty acids increase the amount of oxygen consumed by the heart and decrease its ability to pump blood. This can irritate the muscle of the heart, decreasing its efficiency. If there is already a reduction in blood flow to the heart due to coronary artery disease, then the heart's function may deteriorate even more. Free fatty acids also can induce platelet aggregation, leading to further decreases in coronary blood flow.

Emotional stress also can cause high blood levels of free fatty acids. As described earlier, emotional stress increases the secretion of norepinephrine and epinephrine into the bloodstream; this causes an increase in the breakdown of fat into free fatty acids.

Free fatty acids are an efficient source of energy for running or fighting, so it is useful to have increased amounts of them during times of stress. Unfortunately, when you are chronically stressed and neither fight nor run, you have an *excess* of free fatty acids in your bloodstream—more than your body can use. Likewise, a high-fat diet can result in excessive blood levels of free fatty acids.

What causes fixed blockages to occur in the coronary arteries? Most scientists believe that blockages begin when the inner lining of a coronary artery is chronically injured.

What causes this injury? As you may have guessed by now, high levels of cholesterol in the blood, coronary artery spasm, and stress hormones seem to be the main causes of injuries to the coronary arteries. Cigarette smoking and hypertension are other important causes. Turbulence, caused by obstructions to coronary blood flow, also causes injury.

Let's examine each of these:

Coronary Artery Spasm. The inner lining of the coronary arteries can be damaged when they go into spasm. Chronic stress tends to lead to frequent coronary artery spasm in some people, thus leading to repeated injury to the coronary arteries.

Turbulence. When blood hits the lining of the coronary arteries with excessive force, it can cause injury. This is turbulence. It can be caused in several ways.

For example, when coronary arteries go into spasm, the blood is forced to pass through a narrowed vessel. This can cause turbulence. High blood pressure—which may be caused in many people by chronic stress and a high-fat, high-salt, high-cholesterol diet, among other factors—also causes increased turbulence in blood flow through the coronary arteries. As plaque begins to build up, the blood is forced to pass through an even more narrowed vessel, causing more turbulence—leading to more injury and plaque buildup in a vicious cycle.

Cigarette Smoking. Carbon monoxide, nicotine, tar, and other substances contained in tobacco smoke can injure the lining of the coronary arteries. Since most people who smoke do so throughout the day, the injuries due to smoking are chronic.

Besides causing injury, the carbon monoxide in smoke makes the problem even worse. Oxygen is carried in the blood by molecules called hemoglobin. Carbon monoxide binds so tightly to the hemoglobin that it prevents the blood from carrying oxygen. Since the main problem in coronary heart disease is that the heart is not receiving enough oxygen, you can see why smoking cigarettes is one of the least healthful habits a person can have.

High Levels of Cholesterol in the Blood. The cholesterol in your body comes from two places: you eat it and your body makes it. For most people, high levels of cholesterol in the blood are caused by the cholesterol and the saturated fat that we eat.

When the diet is high in cholesterol, the level of cholesterol in the blood is usually elevated. Too much cholesterol in the blood can injure the lining of the coronary arteries.

Most people in this country eat food that is high in cholesterol at almost every meal. As a result, the blood levels of cholesterol tend to become chronically elevated. This can cause chronic injury to the walls of the coronary arteries. Also, high levels of cholesterol cause the arteries to become more permeable to it. More cholesterol is then absorbed, injuring the arteries still further in a vicious cycle.

As stated earlier, one of the themes of this book is that coronary heart disease is a disease of excess. For example, cholesterol is not "bad"—in fact, your body uses it as the basic building block to manufacture important hormones. But your body makes all the cholesterol that it needs. For most of us, the problem is that there is too much of it in the bloodstream because of the cholesterol we eat, not because of the cholesterol our bodies make. (There are some relatively rare genetic diseases that are exceptions to this.)

Cholesterol is found only in foods of animal origin—meat, chicken, fish, dairy products, and so on. Therefore, if you do not eat animal products, you do not eat cholesterol—it's as simple as that. The average adult American consumes 450 to 600 milligrams of cholesterol a day. In contrast, the participants in our research ate only 5 milligrams of cholesterol a day. (All of it came from the yogurt.)

A large amount of dietary cholesterol not only causes an excessive level of cholesterol in the blood, it also causes the body to produce a substance (a type of lipoprotein) called *beta-VLDL*. This is produced only when the diet is rich in fats and cholesterol.

Dr. Robert W. Mahley, a pathologist at the University of California at San Francisco, demonstrated in 1981 that beta-VLDL delivers cholesterol to scavenger cells called macrophages that line the walls of coronary arteries. Beta-VLDL causes the cholesterol concentration in these cells to rise one hundred to two hundred times the normal level.

Dr. Mahley recently explained that "no beta-VLDL is present in the blood of individuals consuming a low-fat, low-cholesterol diet. In animals, the increase in arterial cholesterol deposits following a fatty diet has been noted in every animal studied. I don't think man would be an exception." This is only one of several means by which high-fat, high-cholesterol diets may cause coronary heart disease. Dr. Joseph Goldstein at the University of Texas Health Science Center found similar evidence.

Not only the amount of fat and cholesterol in the diet are important—the type of *protein* may also be important. Dietary protein seems to have a marked influence on the level of cholesterol in the blood and the development of coronary heart disease. This was first described as early as 1909 by Dr. A. Ignatowski, but once it was shown a few years later that cholesterol could produce heart disease, the role of dietary protein was largely overlooked until recently. According to Dr. K. K. Carroll at the University of Western Ontario (Canada), "The positive correlation between animal protein in the diet and mortality from coronary heart disease is at least as strong as that between dietary fat and heart disease."

In general, animal protein has been found to increase the level of cholesterol in the bloodstream, even in experiments in which the cholesterol and fat have been removed from the protein. However, plant protein does not increase the level of cholesterol. In fact, studies by Dr. Carroll in Canada and by Dr. C. R. Sirtori at the University of Milan (Italy) have shown that vegetable protein may actually *reduce* blood levels of cholesterol (these studies are controversial).

One way that plant protein seems to exert a protective effect is by reducing the absorption of cholesterol from the intestines into the bloodstream. Although plant protein is high in fiber, the effect may be independent of this. The fiber adds additional benefits, including an increased ability to excrete bile acids (which are made from cholesterol). In contrast, animal protein slows the excretion of cholesterol (by reducing the conversion of cholesterol to bile acids), thus allowing blood levels of cholesterol to rise.

Excessive cholesterol not only injures the lining of the coronary arteries, it also provides the building blocks of plaque. Platelets act as the cement. As mentioned earlier, blood platelets are the body's first defense against bleeding. They are the cellular components of the blood that help it to clot.

Platelets circulate in the bloodstream as elliptical flat discs. When the lining of any blood vessel in your body is damaged—as when you cut yourself—platelets are attracted to the site of injury. Here, they become round, develop "false feet" called pseudopods, become sticky, and adhere to the injured area. This forms a plug that repairs the defect and reestablishes the smooth continuity of the blood vessel lining. This is a valuable survival mechanism—it keeps you from bleeding to death whenever you cut yourself.

The same mechanism exists in your coronary arteries. Likewise, this has survival value—platelets help to repair occasional injuries to the lining of your coronary arteries when they occur.

Platelets release substances that cause smooth muscle cells to migrate from the arterial wall to the damaged area, where these cells proliferate. Here, the smooth muscle cells actively absorb cholesterol and fat and secrete fibrous substances. This acts as a type of Band-Aid, which covers the damaged area of the lining. It may take up to nine months for the lining to heal itself.

If further injury does not again stimulate these changes, then the vessel wall may return to normal. However, if the injury is repetitive due to large amounts of cholesterol and fat in the blood or via the other mechanisms described earlier (coronary spasm, emotional stress, cigarette smoking, and so on), then these vessel abnormalities may not regress. Instead, they may degenerate into fixed plaque, obstructing the coronary arteries. This is known as atherosclerosis or arteriosclerosis. In other words, *repetitive* injuries to the coronary arteries cause the repair mechanism of platelets to be destructive rather than lifesaving.

Elevated levels of cholesterol in the blood are caused not only by diet but also by emotional stress. When people are emotionally stressed, the level of cholesterol in the blood rises—independent of diet. The inability to cope with chronic stress can cause a large rise in these levels. On the other hand, stress management training may *reduce* blood levels of cholesterol.

Stress Hormones. As stated earlier, emotional stress can cause the release of the stress hormones norepinephrine and epinephrine. These hormones can cause direct injury to the lining of the coronary arteries. Also, they may injure the coronary arteries by causing coronary artery spasm and platelet clumping to occur.

Another factor besides emotional stress can cause the release of norepinephrine and epinephrine into the bloodstream: caffeine. This stimulant is found not only in coffee, but also in most teas (except some herbal teas such as peppermint), chocolate, cola drinks, and many over-the-counter medications (such as aspirin compounds and nonprescription diet pills). Caffeine also makes irregular heartbeats more likely to occur in many people.

Surprisingly, most people (60 percent) who die from coronary heart disease do not die from heart attacks (myocardial infarction) —they die from what is called, quite appropriately, *sudden cardiac death*.

Sudden cardiac death is the leading cause of mortality in the industrially developed world. In the United States alone, more than 1,200 individuals *each day* die suddenly—approximately one death per minute. Most of these people are in the most productive phase of their lives, seemingly healthy men in their forties and fifties. Sudden cardiac death usually strikes without warning.

The majority of these deaths are the result of sudden, irregular heartbeats which can progress to a disorganized rhythm known as *ventricular fibrillation*. When this happens, the heart is beating so chaotically that it no longer can pump blood effectively. Since the brain can live without blood and oxygen for only a few minutes, death occurs very quickly.

What causes ventricular fibrillation? Emotional stress profoundly increases the occurrence of sudden cardiac death via a series of interactions between the brain and the heart. Dietary factors also seem to play an important role.

Recognition of an association between sudden death and profound emotion dates to the dawn of recorded history. As far back as written records exist, people have been described as dying of cardiovascular disease while experiencing intense fear, rage, grief, humiliation, or joy. In the Bible, when Ananias was charged by Peter, "You have not lied to man but to God," he fell down and died (Acts 5:1-5). Pope Innocent IV succumbed suddenly to the "morbid effects of grief on his system" soon after the disastrous overthrow of his army by Manfred. In the eighteenth century, John Hunter (a noted English physician and surgeon) predicted the manner of his death when he said, "My life is at the mercy of any scoundrel who chooses to put me in a passion." He died in 1793 during an intense debate at a hospital board meeting.

In 1971, Dr. George Engel of the University of Rochester School of Medicine compiled 170 newspaper accounts of sudden cardiac death. Common to all is that they followed events which were impossible for the victim to ignore and to which their responses were overwhelming excitement or despair or both.

Despite this long history of anecdotal evidence, little medical research was conducted into the causes of sudden cardiac death until about ten years ago, and almost no studies examined the possible role of psychological factors. Why not? One reason may be that scientists tend to avoid studying areas in which they do not have the tools to measure what they are observing—even when these areas are very important.

In this context, the following story may be analogous. A man spent several hours on his hands and knees under a streetlamp looking for his missing watch. A passer-by stopped to help. After several hours of looking, he asked in frustration, "Tell me, sir, exactly where did you lose your watch?" The man replied, "Well, I lost it over there in that dark alley, but the light's much better over here."

Yet, as Dr. Engel wrote, "The puzzling fact remains that, with only a little encouragement, many physicians in private conversations are quite ready to recount from their own practices examples of patients who apparently died suddenly under [emotionally charged] circumstances."

Until recently, physicians simply did not know why patients died suddenly. The victim of sudden cardiac death was available only for burial, not for psychological or electro-physiological study. Autopsies showed only some fixed blockages in the coronary arteries, but usually no evidence of heart attacks (infarcted tissue). As a result, sudden cardiac death was puzzling and it was viewed only as the culmination of blockages in the coronary arteries that became progressively worse over a period of many years.

The advent of resuscitative techniques, including cardiopulmonary resuscitation (CPR), made it possible to resuscitate people who were clinically "dead." Continuous electrocardiographic monitoring demonstrated that most of these near-deaths were due to ventricular fibrillation. Subsequent research indicated that the most important mechanisms of sudden cardiac death were short-term and frequently reversible, which raised the exciting possibility that sudden cardiac death may be preventable, at least in some cases.

What are the short-term mechanisms that cause sudden cardiac death due to ventricular fibrillation? As described earlier, emotional stress results in a chronic overstimulation of the sympathetic nervous system; this overstimulation can cause both coronary artery spasm and platelet clumping to occur. Also, a high-fat, high-cholesterol diet can lead to both coronary artery spasm and platelet clumping via other mechanisms previously discussed.

This can cause several things to happen:

Sudden Reduction in Blood Flow to the Heart. The heart seems to be especially vulnerable to rapid changes in coronary blood flow. Besides causing chest pain, sudden decreases in coronary blood flow can cause the heart to beat irregularly, especially when these are followed by sudden increases in coronary blood flow. Both coronary artery spasm and platelet clumping in coronary arteries can cause these transient changes in coronary blood flow.

The heart can adapt to gradual changes in coronary blood flow better than to sudden ones. Ventricular fibrillation is most often caused by a *sudden* change in blood flow to these pacemaker areas of the heart rather than by the gradual reduction in blood flow resulting from the slow buildup of fixed blockages in the coronary arteries.

However, fixed blockages increase the likelihood that ventricular fibrillation may occur. Why? When there are fixed blockages in the coronary arteries, less coronary artery spasm or platelet clumping is required to completely shut off coronary blood flow. Also, turbulent flow in the region of blockages favors the formation of platelet clumping for reasons discussed earlier.

However, if coronary artery spasm or platelet clumping is severe enough, then blood flow can be obstructed even in the absence of fixed blockages. Dr. Bernard Lown reported the case of a thirty-nine-year-old man under substantial emotional stress who had twice experienced ventricular fibrillation even though extensive studies, including coronary angiography, showed no evidence of coronary artery blockage. Dr. Lown also studied forty-three patients who had been resuscitated from ventricular fibrillation or ventricular tachycardia. Eight of these patients had no blockages in their coronary arteries.

Direct Disruption of the Electrical Stability of the Heart. Overstimulation of the sympathetic nervous system due to emotional stress seems to destabilize the heart's conduction system, creating what Dr. Richard Verrier and others have termed an "electrical inhomogeneity" in the heart, causing it to become electrically unstable. In part, this is due to a sudden reduction in coronary blood flow via mechanisms already described. Other neural mechanisms that are not yet fully understood also seem to be involved. When a "critical mass" of the heart is involved, then ventricular fibrillation may occur.

Experiments on laboratory animals by Dr. James Skinner at the Baylor College of Medicine and others have shown that while either a sudden reduction in coronary blood flow or psychological stress can cause ventricular fibrillation to occur, the incidence of this lethal heart rhythm is much higher when both are present. For example, they found that when they suddenly occluded the coronary arteries of pigs (whose hearts are similar to the human heart), the incidence of ventricular fibrillation in an unfamiliar, stressful environment was substantially higher than when coronary artery occlusion was induced in a familiar setting.

The hypothalamus is an area of the brain that is thought to be responsible for the fight-or-flight stress reaction (among other functions). Dr. J. Satinsky and his co-workers at Harvard found that during acute coronary occlusion, stimulation of the sympathetic nervous system and the hypothalamus in anesthetized dogs increased the incidence of ventricular fibrillation tenfold.

In related animal studies by Dr. Lown, Dr. Verrier, and their colleagues at Harvard, just the sight of the experimenter was sometimes enough to produce ventricular fibrillation in dogs who had previously undergone stress-inducing experiments. In a more recent study, Drs. Verrier, Lown, and Federico Lombardi occluded a dog's coronary artery. If the dog was resting when this was done, then he had a small heart attack but did not experience ventricular fibrillation.

They designed an experiment to test whether or not emotional stress would make matters worse. It did. The dog, which had not been fed for the previous twenty-four hours, was allowed to eat only a few bites of food. Another dog was brought in and allowed to eat freely, while the first dog was watching but restrained from eating. Because of this stress, the first dog's heart went into ventricular fibrillation and died. This happened again when they repeated the experiment. Although this study is still ongoing and thus preliminary, it adds further evidence to support the role of psychological stress in causing sudden death.

This appears to be true not only in animals. More than two thousand years ago, Aurelius Cornelius Celsus described the art of taking the pulse:

> When the medical man first comes, the anxiety of the patient, who is in doubt as to what he may seem to him to have, may upset the pulse. For this reason, it is not the part of an experienced doctor that he seize the arm with his hand at once; but first of all sit down with a cheerful expression, and enquire how he feels, and if there is any fear of him, to calm the patient with agreeable talk; and then, at last, lay his hand on the patient's body. How easily a thousand things may disturb the pulse, which even the sight of a doctor may upset!

Unfortunately, Celsus's recommendation is often ignored. In 1955, a study by Dr. K. A. Jarvinen showed that among patients recovering from heart attacks, five times more patients died in conjunction with ward rounds conducted by the chief physician than at other times. The stresses caused by the excitement, anxiety, and disappointments in relation to the patient's progress and discharge from the hospital were considered to be factors in provoking sudden death.

Perhaps the most extreme example of the role of the brain in causing sudden cardiac death due to ventricular fibrillation can be seen in patients who have suffered neurological accidents and are being maintained on life-support systems although legally "brain dead." Because of the lack of higher nervous system input, these patients never experience ventricular fibrillation.

Dr. Lown and his associates also have found that the amount of a chemical in the brain, serotonin, can influence the susceptibility to sudden death. They found that a decrease in brain serotonin increases the risk of sudden death due to ventricular fibrillation, while an increase in brain serotonin decreases the risk of sudden death. Studies by Dr. Richard Wurtman, Professor of Neuroendocrine Regulation at the Massachusetts Institute of Technology, have demonstrated that the type of diet influences the amount of brain serotonin. In particular, diets that are high in carbohydrate (like Groups 1 and 2) cause an increase in serotonin; this may reduce the risk of sudden death, all other things being equal. It is as if the amount of sympathetic stimulation to the heart were reduced. Conversely, diets that are high in protein (like the typical American diet) seem to reduce the amount of brain serotonin, and this probably increases the risk of sudden death. (The mechanism seems to involve the ratio of tryptophan to the other essential amino acids.) This work is preliminary but very exciting.

Studies of large groups of people indicate that there is an increased prevalence of sudden death during bereavement or following significant life changes. In the first six months after the loss of a spouse, the death rate among widows and widowers increased 40 percent above the expected rate. Dr. R. H. Rahe interviewed the families of 226 victims of sudden cardiac death and noted that significant life changes such as divorce, grief, and altered work patterns had occurred during the six months preceding death compared with the same interval one year earlier. Other studies have shown that the incidence of sudden death is much higher on Monday (when the stresses of returning to work are high) than on other days of the week.

In a study conducted in 1981, Dr. Regis A. DeSilva (another associate of Dr. Lown) and Dr. Peter Reich interviewed 117 patients who were admitted following emergency resuscitation for ventricular fibrillation or other serious rhythm disorders. Twenty-five of these patients reported that a serious interpersonal conflict had taken place in the twenty-four hours before their life-threatening attacks. The emotional episodes included on-the-job conflicts, violent family fights, and a variety of other disturbing situations. In one instance, a Yankee fan suffered ventricular fibrillation as he watched his team lose an exciting game to the Red Sox.

In a letter to the *New England Journal of Medicine*, Dr. Thomas Graboys of the Brigham and Women's Hospital in Boston described a patient of his, an avid Boston Celtics fan, who underwent twenty-four-hour electrocardiographic monitoring while watching the Celtics in an exciting playoff game on television. As the game progressed, the frequency of irregular heartbeats increased, and the type of irregular beats became more pathological. During the final hour of the game (which the Celtics won by only one point), the patient had five episodes of ventricular tachycardia, in many cases a precursor to ventricular fibrillation. The Celtics victory was followed by a gradual decrease in irregular beats over the next two hours.

Does this mean that we should all just sit around, "not get too excited," and lead boring lives? No. In the next chapter, I will discuss how emotional stress is caused primarily by our *perception* of the environment and our reactions to it—not just by the environment itself.

In conclusion, coronary heart disease is in many respects a disease of excess—harmful reactions to chronic stresses and a diet based on excessive animal products. These appear to chronically activate the web of mechanisms described in this chapter, which in turn may reduce coronary blood flow and lead to the manifestations of coronary heart disease: chest pain (angina), heart attack, or sudden cardiac death.

On the next page is a diagram that summarizes all of the mechanisms described in this chapter. While it appears ridiculously complex, I include it primarily to illustrate that all of these mechanisms interrelate. Therefore, a combined program that simultaneously addresses as many of these mechanisms as possible is likely to result in the most rapid improvements (and to have the best potential for reducing the risk of developing coronary heart disease).

Our program is based on a simple concept—removing the excesses that may lead to coronary heart disease. Foods in Group 1 of the diet are very low in fat and contain no cholesterol. The

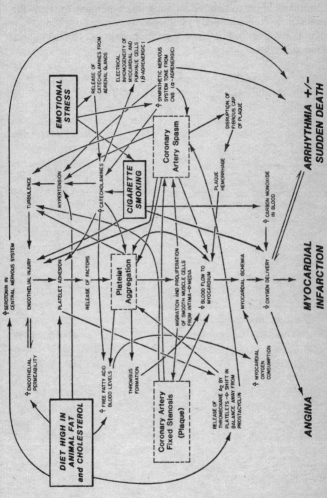

Figure 5. This diagram shows the web of mechanisms that cause coronary heart disease.

program describes how to react to stress in ways that are less harmful and how to remove physical and emotional tension when they occur. It is designed to help you increase your productivity and enjoyment—while reducing your risk of coronary heart disease.

5. Assumptions: Why Do We Feel Stressed?

"My crown is in my heart, not on my head;
not decked with diamonds and Indian stones, nor to be seen;
my crown is called content;
a crown it is that seldom kings enjoy."
—WILLIAM SHAKESPEARE, *Henry VI, Part III*

"ever
ybody
wants more
(&more &
still More) what the
hell are we all morticians?"
—E. E. CUMMINGS, *95 Poems*

Look around. In almost every type of job, at almost every level of employment, you can see driven, stressed, alienated, unhappy people. Why? What causes emotional stress?

This chapter, unlike the previous ones, is derived primarily from my experiences rather than from objectively verifiable data or the work of others. It describes the assumptions upon which the program is based.

We are used to thinking of emotional stress as coming from outside ourselves. Certainly, most of us view some situations as being inherently stressful—asking the boss for a raise, giving a public lecture, and so on.

Yet it is primarily our *reaction* to a stressful situation that is harmful, not simply the situation itself. Two people who are faced with the same event may activate the fight-or-flight response in varying degrees—one may become quite stressed, while the other may hardly feel stressed at all.

For example, air traffic controllers have highly stressful jobs.

Because of this, most doctors believed that they would be likely to develop stress-related illnesses. However, Dr. Robert Rose (University of Texas Medical School) studied 416 air traffic controllers for three years. He found that the incidence of illness, both physical and psychiatric, was directly related to the attitude the men had to their work. In other words, *the intensity of the stress was less important than the way it was perceived.*

Similarly, a few years after he returned from the moon, one of the astronauts said, "Life in the business world has been much more stressful than anything I did during the space program." It might be assumed that being blasted into space and traveling to the moon would be one of life's more stressful experiences. Yet even though this environment was quite hostile, the astronaut had been trained in simulations, over and over, to react to it in a healthy way.

The implication of these examples is important. If we view a situation as being inherently stressful, then we are powerless to do anything about it (except to avoid all stress, which is impossible—and not even desirable). On the other hand, if stress is caused primarily by our reactions to situations, then we have the power to learn to react in ways that are healthful rather than harmful.

What determines whether or not we react to situations in ways that are stressful? We know that there is a common response to stress—the fight-or-flight reaction. Is there a common reason why we perceive situations as being stressful?

I believe that there is. Listen to two of the participants in our study:

> Even though I have been successful at most things I've done in my life, each time I was doing something I just looked forward to completing it. I always wanted something else to happen. But when it did, I felt deflated rather than elated. I've lived most of my life that way. I recall always wanting to get out of high school because then I was really going to be happy. Then I couldn't wait to get out of college, and next I wanted to complete pilot training. I looked forward to reaching my goals, but the anticipation was always sweeter than the realization. The first time I made a thousand dollars, or the first time I made a hundred thousand, or the first time

I did anything, it was as much of a letdown as the anticipation and realization of any other goal. To compensate for that letdown and boredom, I started setting three and four goals at the same time. I gave up on the word "happy" and replaced it with "self-satisfaction." In my mind, "happiness" goes with a small child or an adult with a diminished I.Q.
                                                                    —TED G., a prominent stockbroker

When I am doing a job, most of the time there is more at stake than just getting the work done. My sense of self-worth is usually involved—I'm afraid that I won't measure up. For example, when I was working for the telephone company as a service representative, we had such a workload that there was no way that one person could finish all the work I was assigned to do in one day. At the time, I was naïve enough to think that the phone company had ways of estimating how much work a person should be able to do in a day's time, and that if the work was there to be done then I should be able to finish it by the end of the day. When I couldn't do it all, I got very, very upset. I felt like I was not measuring up because I couldn't do all that there was to do. I began to believe that I was not as good as the other representatives there. I do this all the time. When I make a mistake, it shatters me. Even if everybody is nice about it and says, "Well, we all make mistakes," I still can't stand it. It causes a turmoil inside of me because I just don't make any allowances for mistakes. I am more tolerant of other people's mistakes than of my own. If I fail at doing something, I feel like I'm a failure as a person.
                                                                    —ELLEN W., retired service representative

These two statements seem to be completely opposite. Ted believes that he can accomplish whatever he sets out to achieve, but he is dissatisfied because reaching his goals never seems to bring him more than temporary pleasure. Ellen believes that whatever she accomplishes is not good enough, so she often views herself as a failure. Ted searches for contentment from his achievements; Ellen looks for hers in the approval of others.

Yet despite these seeming differences, when we look beneath the surface we find that there is a common reason why Ted and

Ellen feel stressed: they see themselves as lacking, and they identify—actually, they *mis*-identify—something or someone that they believe will bring them lasting contentment.

To one extent or another, almost all of us do this because we often feel that we are lacking something or someone. We tell ourselves, "If only I had————, then I would be content," and we fill in this blank with power, sex, money, prestige, someone's love, achievements, approval, material wealth, and endless variations on these themes.

This is where stress usually begins. Once we have made this mis-identification, we usually feel stressed no matter what happens.

If we don't get what we want, of course, we are disappointed and stressed.

Until we get what we want, we feel stressed. We may have a pleasurable feeling of anticipation, but there is usually anxiety and fear as well: "Am I going to get what I want? What if I don't? What if somebody else gets it instead?" Or, as Ellen asked, "Will I measure up?"

Even if we get what we want, we still lose—that is, we feel stressed—in several ways.

First, it is never enough: *Now what*? As Ted said, "Each time I was doing something I just looked forward to completing it. . . . To compensate for that letdown and boredom, I started setting three and four goals at the same time."

Barbara J., another participant, also was successful at most of what she attempted. "I was always the one they picked to be the leader, the president of this or the chairman of that. But I was always left with a restless feeling: 'Is this all there is?' "

One man expressed it this way when he first entered our study: "I can't even enjoy the view from the mountain I've climbed, because I'm already looking over at the next mountain. The more I get, the more I want."

Second, getting what we want usually does not bring the lasting contentment that we expected: *So what*? "Big deal." Ted's comment was representative of many: "The anticipation was always sweeter than the realization."

Third, even after we've gotten what we want, we often feel anxiety and fear—more stress. "Will I lose what I have attained? Will someone take it away from me? How can I protect it?" So we construct barriers, literally and figuratively, to protect what we have accumulated. This further isolates us, reinforcing our belief that we are lacking.

Yet we rarely ask ourselves, "Why do I feel dissatisfied and unfulfilled so often? What is the underlying cause of the stress that I feel?" The momentary satisfaction that comes from getting what we want seduces us into believing that we can get lasting contentment from "out there."

So we usually make the same mistake again: "Well, *this* didn't bring me a lasting sense of contentment—but maybe *that* will." In other words, we mis-identify again. We look in the wrong place. In this way, we establish another stress cycle. For many of us, this treadmill is a way of life. (In this context, it is perhaps an appropriate metaphor that most heart patients find themselves running on a treadmill as part of their diagnostic evaluation.)

Because we view ourselves as lacking, we try to fill the perceived emptiness with excess. We continually drive ourselves in an attempt to satisfy the void that we feel. As we have seen, it is excesses of food and stress that may lead to coronary heart disease. Ironically, coronary heart disease seems to be a disease of excess caused by our perception that we are lacking.

Of course, we feel good when we get what we want—but it never seems to last, for the reasons described earlier. Is it possible to feel a lasting sense of contentment?

Perhaps so. If contentment is based only on getting what we want, then it is only temporary. But contentment is primarily an *inner* process, not something we can get.

Unfortunately, we almost never give ourselves a chance to feel at ease—we are always running after what we think will bring us contentment, continually adding more stress. In other words, in the process of striving to get what we think will bring us contentment, we paradoxically disturb the well-being that we could already have.

It may seem as though contentment is the result of getting what we want. When we get what we want, we stop for a moment and allow ourselves to feel content—at least for a while, we are no longer disturbing our inner sense of contentment by chasing after something or someone. But we then attribute this feeling to getting what we thought we needed rather than simply to having stilled the disturbances for a moment. So we run after something or someone else, and the feelings of stress begin again.

The Program

We cannot break free of this stress cycle simply by learning how to cope with stress better, how to avoid it, or how to use new behavioral modification techniques to "deal" with it more effectively. The easiest way to stop reacting to situations in stressful ways is to experience an inner contentment.

The program described in this book is one way of enabling us to do this. The techniques that are described in Part Two do not *bring* contentment. They simply help to identify and remove disturbances that keep us from feeling at ease. For example, at the end of a progressive deep relaxation (page 96), remind yourself that your increased sense of well-being did not come from getting what you thought you needed, but rather from simply removing whatever was disturbing what you already had.

To summarize what we have discussed so far: because we usually feel lacking, we mis-identify something or someone "out there" as being able to bring us a lasting sense of well-being. In the process of striving to get this, ironically, we disturb our inner contentment.

In the final analysis, we feel stress primarily because of how we perceive the world. Our behaviors are a result of our motivations. Our motivations, in turn, are a result of how we perceive the world and ourselves. Therefore, it is not sufficient only to change behaviors; it is necessary to change our perceptions.

As discussed, we misperceive ourselves as lacking. This, in turn, is the result of a more basic misperception: seeing ourselves as being fundamentally separate from everyone and everything else—that is, *apart from* the world rather than *a part of* it. Isolated and fragmented. Cut off. Alone.

In this context, there seem to be two kinds of perceptions (and thus two primary motivations): those that tend to erect barriers that reinforce the idea of separateness and lacking (leading to stress and eventually to disease), and those that help to break through these barriers (leading to contentment and health).

For example, in our two cardiovascular research studies, the participants were a diverse group. They came from a wide spectrum of socioeconomic and educational backgrounds and ranged from a large company's president to a man who could not even afford his cardiac medications, from a person with several graduate degrees to one who had never finished the third grade.

In each study, the participants lived together for several weeks.

On the first day, most were acutely aware of their differences. After a few days, though, it became apparent that they had much more in common than they had previously thought. People who ordinarily would not have spent much time together now found that their responses to having a life-threatening illness were remarkably similar. Instead of setting themselves apart from each other, they began to help one another, making an effort to understand and to share feelings with each other that they usually would have kept to themselves. Beneath the seeming differences, they shared many of the same hopes and fears and were grappling with similar problems.

In other words, the boundaries that had separated them from each other—and from themselves—began to crumble somewhat. To a large degree, I believe that this contributed to the beneficial cardiovascular results that we later measured.

This is not really so farfetched or simplistic. A study by Dr. Robert Nerem reported in *Science* magazine (1980) demonstrated that rabbits on a high-cholesterol diet that were petted, handled, talked to, and played with showed more than a 60 percent reduction in the degree of blockage in their coronary arteries when compared to an otherwise identical group of rabbits that were given the same diet. This was true even though serum cholesterol levels, heart rate, and blood pressure were comparable in both groups.

Other studies have indicated that the counterpart also may be true: people who have pets tend to have a lower incidence of sudden cardiac death than those who live alone. Having a pet—or being petted—may help to break through a perceived sense of isolation.

Similarly, in the 1960s, Drs. Stewart Wolf and Helen Goodell found that rural Italians living in the Roseto community in Pennsylvania had a low death rate from coronary heart disease even though their diet was rich in fat and cholesterol. Why? Their families were stable, closely knit, and relatively secure, with strong community ties. With increasing urbanization and disruption of the family, the sudden death rates increased and are now approaching those of adjoining communities.

Throughout the history of medicine doctors have considered the idea that close relationships to other people have a beneficial effect on health, but it is only in the past two decades that this concept has had any scientific documentation. Several studies indicate that close relationships are important to maintaining good health.

For example, Dr. James J. Lynch found that in 225 patients in a coronary care unit, a significant reduction in ventricular arrhythmias (irregular heartbeats) occurred simply when the doctor or nurse touched the patient long enough to take the pulse. His book, *The Broken Heart*, surveys the scientific literature in this area and makes a convincing point that social isolation contributes to causing coronary heart disease.

Unfortunately, much of what we do in our society—and in most industrialized societies—tends to reinforce the differences between us rather than the similarities. We categorize entire groups of people by race, heritage, country, religion, sex, social class, schools attended—a thousand and one ways to set ourselves apart from others. As a teacher once told me, "We are all born 'fine.' Around the age of two, we get 'educated' and we begin to *de-fine* ourselves: 'I'm white, I'm an American, I'm a male,' and so on, and we get caught in these definitions."

Somehow, we believe that by setting ourselves apart, we can gain love and intimacy—another paradox. "Look at me, I'm special—I have this, and I've done that." We sometimes think that by accentuating the differences between us, we can break down the barriers that separate us—yet this only reinforces the isolation that we feel.

Of course, this does not mean that we should all be alike. Definitions can allow us to enjoy life's diversity—but too often they are used to reinforce our sense of isolation and separation.

As mentioned in Chapter 3, Drs. Friedman and Rosenman found that what they called "Type A behavior," characterized by ambitiousness, competitiveness, and a sense of time urgency, is associated with an increased risk of developing coronary heart disease. But these behavioral traits are not *causes* of coronary heart disease; rather, they are *symptoms* of ways of viewing the world which may lead to coronary heart disease.

That is, if you see yourself as fundamentally lacking and separate and you believe, "If only I had————, I'd be happy," then ambitiousness, competitiveness, and time urgency logically follow. "The more I get, the happier I'll be. The more other people get, the less there is for me. If someone else gets happier, then I'll be sadder. I can't waste time relaxing—I'll be missing a chance to get more. This is a dog-eat-dog world." Finally, the heart whispers, "You can stop now."

Dr. Larry Scherwitz, one of the principal co-investigators of our studies, further refined Friedman and Rosenman's work. He found that Type A people used personal pronouns in their speech—I, me, my, mine—twice as frequently as those who were Type B. Furthermore, he found that those who used these words frequently in their conversation were much more likely to have abnormal electrocardiograms than those who used these self-references less frequently.

In another study, Dr. Scherwitz and his colleagues interviewed 150 men before coronary angiography. They found that the more frequently patients referred to themselves (I, me, my, mine) during the interview, the more severe was their coronary artery disease and the more likely that they had suffered an earlier heart attack. Furthermore, men who used frequent self-references tended to have lower exercise tolerance (on a treadmill) and a lower cardiac ejection fraction. Self-references remained a signficant correlate of the extent of disease, even when controlled for age, blood pressure, cholesterol, and Type A behavior. In her dissertation, Dr. Linda Powell found self-references to predict future recurrent heart attacks (myocardial infarctions) even when controlled for Type A and other behaviors.

Why? This exaggerated focus on the self may further reinforce the sense of isolation and separateness. Frequent use of these self-pronouns seems to indicate a strong sense of perceived separateness.

If lasting contentment is not to be found in the external world, does that mean we should sit around and contemplate our navels? Of course not. If we focus our awareness internally, doesn't this just intensify our sense of isolation? I don't think so.

To be content does not mean to be passive. To be peaceful does not mean to be lazy. We can accomplish a lot when we are feeling at ease. Paradoxically, the more content we are, the more assertive and productive we can be both to ourselves and for others. Anxiety interferes with being productive, and fear inter- feres with being assertive.

Moreover, the more content we are, the less we feel the need to manipulate others to get what we think we need. Other people are then viewed as less threatening to our well-being. As a result, our relationships tend to become heathier and the barriers that separate and isolate us tend to fall away. In the final analysis, this is a position of strength: if contentment is primarily an inner process, then it is also true that no one can take this feeling away unless we allow them to do so.

I am not suggesting that we should selfishly withdraw from the world; rather, this is a way of learning how we can live more effectively and usefully in it. This is not a "Me Generation" or "Looking out for Number One" approach. If anything, the opposite is true. By taking a few minutes each day to remove tension and to experience an inner sense of well-being, you will be more peaceful and useful to others—while feeling better in the process. Of course, you must first take care of yourself before you can be useful to others—even the heart pumps blood to itself first. It is difficult to accomplish very much when you are in pain or in a hospital bed.

The goal of our program is not just to live longer or to lose weight or even to reduce heart disease, desirable though these may be. It is to become more free of the self-imposed limitations that we erect and to help break through the boundaries that separate us from each other and from ourselves.

I do not pretend to have made much progress—just a few faltering steps. I still feel stressed—more often than not, but less than I used to. I don't get chest pain but may become anxious, angry, worried, or depressed from time to time. In this context, almost all of us have "diseases of the heart." But at least I usually can make the connection between when I feel stressed and why. The pain is the first step toward the solution. Rather than blame someone else, I can usually attribute the stress to my misperceptions—"If only I had————, then I'd be happy." When this happens, I gently remind myself, "Well, you blew it again."

Once this connection has been made, it becomes easier to begin changing the perceptions which cause us to feel this way. That is, the stress teaches us that there are less painful ways of viewing the world—and each time, it gets a little easier.

Part Two
STRESS MANAGEMENT TECHNIQUES

"As a man thinketh in his heart, so is he."

—Proverbs 23:7

"Man is what he believes."

—ANTON CHEKHOV

"Sometimes I've believed as many as six impossible things before breakfast."

—LEWIS CARROLL

What follows is a step-by-step handbook that will show you the program. All of the various components interrelate. For simplicity, however, the handbook is divided into two major sections: (1) the stress management techniques and (2) the diet.

This handbook is simply a guide, not a perscription. As stated in the Introduction, all this book can do is to show you what I have learned. Judge for yourself how much of it is useful to you. While most of the patients who participated in our research followed the program in its entirety, you may find that some aspects of it are more appealing and useful than others. The program is a spectrum, not all or nothing.

We are all different; no program can be designed to meet the needs of everyone. You may want to adapt some aspects of the program to better suit you, or you may want to use the information here to design your own program. You are the final authority on what is right for you.

The unifying purpose of the program's different elements is to enable you to gain progressively more awareness and control over your body and mind. (Learning to stand on your own two feet is much more important than learning to stand on your head.) Increasing self-awareness is the key to this program. Before you can solve a problem, of course, you first have to know what it is. For example, you have to know what is stressful to you before you can learn to deal with it more effectively or to prevent it from happening.

This program is simple to learn and easy to do. These are new skills, so they may take time to master—but even a little practice may yield impressive results. Of course, as with any skill, the more you practice, the better you become at doing it and the more enjoyable it becomes.

Keep in mind that the purpose of the techniques described in this handbook is not just to lower your blood pressure or your cholesterol, or even to help you live longer—although it may help you to do all of these. It is to feel freer and to more fully enjoy life now.

This handbook can help to reintroduce you to two old friends: your body and your mind.

6. Getting Ready

"The time to relax is when you don't have time for it."
—SYDNEY J. HARRIS

It is best to keep your eyes closed while you are practicing these techniques. This will help to keep you focused on what you are doing and on how your body is responding. Of course, you will not be able to read much further with your eyes closed, so . . .

The easiest way to learn this program is either to have someone else read each section aloud while you are doing it or to make a tape for yourself and play it back. It is best to read the entire handbook before beginning to practice any of the techniques in it.

Allow yourself enough time. It is better to do only a few of the techniques with adequate time than to rush through them all—it is difficult to "hurry up and relax." Just do whatever you have time for.

If you have coronary heart disease and you feel any chest discomfort or pain (angina), then lie down immediately until it subsides. Listen to what your heart is telling you, and take it easy for a while.

7. Stretching

This section shows you how to stretch.

Please remember that increasing the awareness of your body and mind is the purpose of everything that follows. As your awareness increases, so does your control. In the process, you will feel more relaxed and peaceful.

We will begin with stretching, since it is much easier to control the body than the mind.

Stretching helps you get to know yourself and how your body feels. As you stretch the various parts, you not only become more flexible, you increase your awareness of them. (Later, in the section on meditation, these principles of self-awareness and flexibility will be extended to include your thoughts and emotions.) Stretching with awareness is the beginning of meditation.

Though simple, these stretches are quite powerful. When done incorrectly, they can do much more harm than good. So be careful.

Most of us have learned several misconceptions about how to stretch: "The farther you can stretch, the better." "The best way to stretch is to bounce up and down." "A good stretch should hurt—no pain, no gain."

Not so. Stretching feels good when done correctly. It is peaceful and relaxing. Like most things in nature, slow and gentle changes are the least stressful.

Here are some basic concepts to keep in mind:

1. The best way to stretch is without bouncing. Whenever you bounce, you may stretch your muscle fibers too far. This activates what is called the "stretch reflex."

Whenever your muscle fibers are stretched too much, they send a signal to the brain: "Help—I can't go this far!" Without having to consciously think about it, your brain automatically responds by sending a nerve impulse that causes these muscle fibers to contract strongly. So, stretching too far paradoxically tightens the muscles which you are trying to relax.

Sometimes, this reflex can help to keep your muscles and joints from being injured. However, the vigorous momentum of bouncing can cause the stretch to continue even while the muscle fibers are contracting—and this can produce damage.

When muscle fibers are injured in this way, it can lead to the formation of scar tissue within them. If the injuries are repeated over a period of time, this causes the fibers to become less elastic—making them even more rigid, rather than more flexible.

A stretch is a stretch is a stretch—it is not a strain.

2. *Take it easy.* These stretches are not calisthenics, and they are not competitions, either with others or with yourself. As explained above, it is not a good idea to stretch too far. When in doubt, do less than your limit. In the beginning, only stretch about half as far as you are able. Once your body realizes that you are not going to hurt it, it will relax even further. Hold the position only as long as it feels comfortable for you.

3. *Think about the areas being stretched.* You will benefit most from these stretches if you pay attention to the parts of your body that you are stretching and experience the changes that are occurring there. With practice, you will become more aware of the messages your body is giving you. Therefore, you will be much less likely to overdo and possibly hurt yourself.

Your body changes from day to day and throughout the day. For example, just because you were able to stretch to a certain point on one day does not necessarily mean that you can do so on the next. (Most people find that they are more limber later in the day.)

4. *Each movement should be slow, fluid, and controlled,* as in ballet rather than calisthenics. (Many of these stretches are similar to those used by dancers.)

5. *Inhale as you stretch backward; exhale when you bend forward.* Breathe slowly and deeply (always through your nose). Try not to hold your breath. If you are not able to breathe easily, then you are stretching too far.

6. *Continue breathing* during the stretch. This will allow your body to relax even further.

7. *Wait a few hours after eating* before you begin these stretches. Any physical movement will divert blood from your digestive system.

8. *Wear loose, comfortable clothing* that will allow your body to move. Also, remove your shoes before you begin.

9. *It is best to keep your eyes closed* while you are doing these exercises, as mentioned before. This will help to keep your awareness focused on what you are doing and on how your body is responding. (Of course, open your eyes if you have trouble maintaining your balance.)

10. *The process is important, not just the goal.* We tend to believe the opposite—that only the goal is important. Instead, approach the stretches as if you were making music or dancing. Making music is not done simply to reach the end of the composition. If that were the purpose, then the fastest players would be the best. Likewise, the purpose of dancing is not to arrive at a specific place on the dance floor. (We will explore this concept in more depth in Chapter 10.)

Remember, the goal is not to see how far you can stretch—what is important is simply to enjoy the process of stretching.

WARMING UP

Before you begin stretching, take a "mental inventory" of how you are doing. Although you may find it tempting to skip this part and get on with the action, remember that increasing the awareness of your body and mind is the basic purpose of everything that follows.

In this exercise you will become more aware of each part of your body, starting with your feet and ending with your head. To begin the inventory, stand with your feet about a shoulder-width apart, with your hands by your side and your eyes closed. (The reason for keeping your eyes closed, of course, is to keep your awareness inward—there are too many interesting distractions out there.)

Begin by becoming aware of your feet and how they feel. Notice where they are tense and recall how they got that way. Ask these parts of your body to let go of some of the tension that they are holding, and allow them to relax somewhat.

Remember that you do not have to *do* anything to remove tension. Trying to force tension out only creates more of it. Just let go of it. You are *allowing* relaxation to occur; you cannot make it happen.

Next, repeat the same process with your ankles. Then, move up your body part by part—calves, knees, thighs, pelvic muscles, lower back, abdominal muscles, upper back, chest, shoulders, arms, hands, neck, face (including the jaw), and head—doing the same thing.

When you've finished, just observe your breathing for a few minutes. Feel the air as it comes in and out of your nose. When your mind wanders—as it will—and you begin to think of all the things that you "should" be doing, or forgot to do, or "shouldn't" have done, gently but firmly bring your awareness back to your breathing. That's all there is to it.

Start with some simple movements:

HEAD ROTATIONS

In this exercise you'll be rolling your head in a circle. It will help to relax your neck muscles and to relieve tension in them. The movement should be slow and gentle, without strain. Throughout the exercise, notice how your neck muscles feel as you rotate your head.

Begin by bringing your awareness to your neck. Then, in a continuous movement, slowly rotate your head in a full circle, giving your neck a gentle stretch at each point along the way. Allow your neck to relax as you do this. First, roll your head slowly in a clockwise direction, then stop and go in the opposite direction a few times. Do not snap your head.

Only take yourself to the point where you feel a mild stretch. If you feel *any* pain at all—even mild discomfort—you are overdoing it. Remember, stretching feels good when it is done correctly.

SHOULDER SHRUGS

Now, bring your head back to the center. First, raise your shoulders up as far as you can without straining. Hold them there for a few seconds, and then slowly bring them down. Do this two or three times.

Rest for a few seconds, and notice how this feels.

Then, rotate your right shoulder in a circular motion—first forward, then backward—feeling a mild stretch along each point of the circle as you do this. Next, do the same with your left shoulder. Allow your shoulders and neck muscles to relax while you are doing this. Now rotate both shoulders together a few times.

BODY TWISTS

Extend your arms away from your sides as you raise them to shoulder level. (Your arms now should be parallel to the floor and perpendicular to your body.) Keeping your arms outstretched, bend them at the elbows.

Now, slowly twist your body at the waist from side to side, feeling a gentle stretch as you do so. Do this a few times. As always, be careful not to overdo it.

At this point, you may wish to rest. So, this is a good time to learn the Resting Position—one of the simplest, yet most effective, of the stress management techniques.

RESTING POSITION

Lie on your back on a mat, blanket, carpet, or thick towel. Place your feet about eighteen inches apart. Let your legs and feet relax so that they are in a comfortable position. Place your arms slightly away from your body, with your palms turned up. If you feel any discomfort in your lower back, place a pillow (or two) under the backs of your knees.

Observe your breath as it flows in and out. When your mind wanders, return your awareness to observing your breathing.

In his research studies, Dr. K. K. Datey documented that the Resting Position produced a substantial and significant reduction

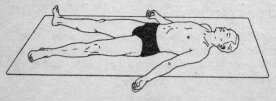

in blood pressure in a group of patients with high blood pressure. Dr. Chandra Patel and others have found it to be similarly useful in their studies.

Now, at last, we can begin to stretch. The first of these—the Twelve-Part Movement—is actually a combination of several stretches.

TWELVE-PART MOVEMENT

This series of movements is particularly valuable because it incorporates many of the benefits of the individual stretches—yet it takes only a few minutes to do.

It is also an excellent warm-up before the individual stretches or before walking, jogging, swimming, bicycling, or other aerobic exercises.

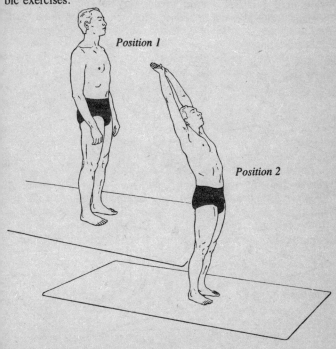

Position 1

Position 2

The Twelve-Part Movement stretches virtually all of your muscle groups, both forward and backward. The movement is divided into twelve separate parts for teaching purposes; however, it is designed to be done in one continuous flow.

Position One. Stand erect (but relaxed) with your eyes closed, your arms by your sides, and your feet about a shoulder-width apart. Briefly repeat the "mental inventory" described earlier.

Position Two. Bring your hands together, locking your thumbs. Slowly extend your arms as far as you can in front of you. Inhale as you begin to slowly raise your arms over your head.

When your arms are extended straight over your head, begin to bend backward—first with your head and then with your torso. Look upward at your hands.

Position Three. Keeping your head between your arms, and your hands together, exhale slowly as you bend forward from the waist until you feel a mild stretch. Try to keep your knees straight. Remember not to bounce. Hold this position for at least

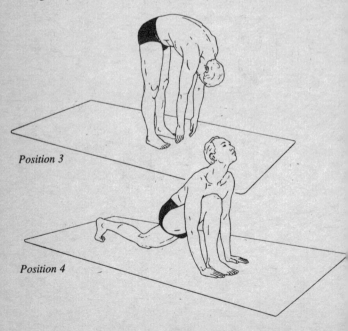

Position 3

Position 4

a few seconds as you continue to slowly inhale and exhale. Let your neck and back muscles relax, simply allowing the weight of your body to gently pull you forward.

Position Four. Now, inhale as you bend your knees. Place each hand on either side of your feet. Keep your right foot where it is (between your hands) and shift your weight to it. Bring your left leg straight back, allowing the left knee to touch the ground. Slowly raise your head as you look up, giving a gentle, pleasant stretch to your back and chest.

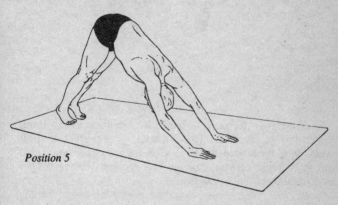

Position 5

Position Five. Bring your right foot back and place it alongside your left foot. Exhale slowly as you push yourself up into a triangle, with your head between your arms, looking back at your feet, feeling a nice stretch in the back of your legs. (If you try to lower your heels toward the floor, you will stretch even more.)

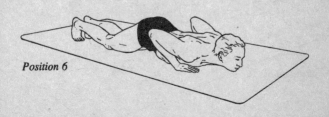

Position 6

Position Six. Shift forward between your arms and inhale slowly as you bring your knees, chest, and chin to the ground—in that order—keeping your pelvis slightly off the floor. (Your hands are by your shoulders, as if you are doing a pushup.)

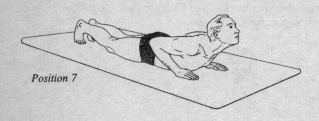

Position 7

Position Seven. Retain your breath for a moment as you lower your pelvis to the floor. Now, transfer your weight to your hands, look up toward the ceiling, and slowly raise your chin and upper chest off the floor as you resume inhaling. (Your pelvis should remain on the floor.)

(*Note*: Now, you are more than halfway through—and there is nothing new to learn. The remaining positions simply repeat the first five, but in the opposite order.)

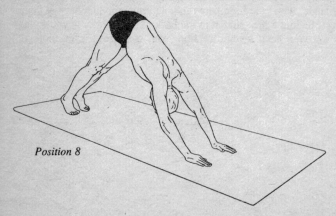

Position 8

Position Eight (same as Position Five). Exhale slowly as you push yourself up into a triangle, with your head between your arms, looking back at your feet. (Your feet should remain about a shoulder-width apart.)

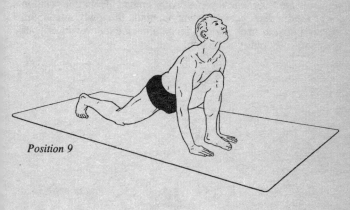

Position 9

Position Nine (similar to Position Four, but with the right leg back). Now, inhale, as you bring your left foot forward, placing it between your hands. (If you need a little help, reach back and gently pull your foot forward.) Allow your right knee to touch the ground. Slowly raise your head as you look up, giving a mild stretch to your back and chest.

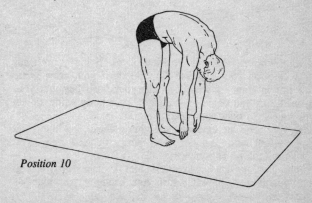

Position 10

Position Ten (same as Position Three). Now, bring your right foot alongside your left foot, keeping your hands on either side of your feet. Straighten your knees, exhale slowly, and bend forward. Remember not to bounce. (Your hands will probably come off the floor unless you are very limber.) Hold this position for at least a few seconds as you continue to slowly inhale and exhale. Let your neck muscles relax, allowing the weight of your body to gently pull you forward.

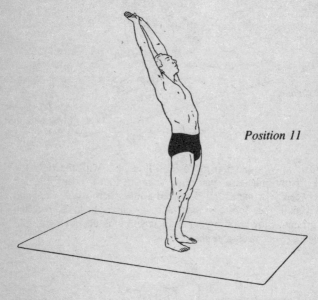

Position 11

Position Eleven (same as Position Two). Bring your hands together, locking your thumbs. Slowly extend your arms as far as you can in front of you. Keeping your head between your arms, inhale as you begin to straighten your body while slowly raising your arms over your head.

When your arms are extended straight overhead, begin to bend backward—first with your head and then with your torso. You may wish to look up at your hands.

Position Twelve (same as Position One). Exhale slowly as you unlock your thumbs. Slowly return your hands to your sides as you stand erect.

* * *

Now, briefly repeat the mental inventory. How do you feel? If you stretched the right amount, you should feel noticeably more relaxed. If you feel any pain, then you overdid it. Repeat the Twelve-Part Movement once or twice again, depending on how you feel.

The next section describes the individual stretches.

BACK STRETCH

Lie on your back in the resting position. For a few moments, breathe slowly and deeply, focusing your attention on your breathing. Feel the rise and fall of your abdomen and chest as you inhale and exhale.

Now, roll over onto your stomach, placing your arms by your sides and your feet slightly apart. Turn your head to one side and relax in this position, keeping your awareness focused on your breathing.

Bring your feet together and place your hands (palms down) on either side of your shoulders, as if you were going to do a pushup. Turn your head back so that your forehead or chin rests on the floor. Inhale slowly and raise your head until you feel a gentle stretch in your neck.

Now, transfer your weight to your hands as you slowly raise your upper chest off the floor. Even though some of your weight is on your hands, allow the muscles of your upper back to do most of the work. (The lower part of your body, from your navel to your toes, should remain on the floor.) Look up as far as you can without straining.

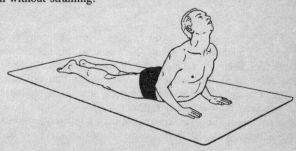

Stay in this position for as long as you feel comfortable (but never longer than a minute), continuing to breathe slowly and deeply. When you are ready, exhale as you slowly come down, lowering first your chest, then your head, to the ground.

Turn your head to the side, bring your arms down along your side (palms up), and place your feet slightly apart. Relax in this Resting Position. Take a moment to see how your back feels. If there is any discomfort, you may have pushed a little too far.

Repeat the stretch once again if you wish.

LEG LIFTS

From the Resting Position (on your front), turn your head back so that your chin rests on the floor. Tuck your arms underneath your thighs with your palms upward. Try to push your elbows close together, but only as far as it is comfortable. Breathe in deeply and hold your breath for just a moment. Straighten your right leg, point your toe, and without bending your knee raise your right leg off the ground as high as you can without straining. Allow your entire weight to rest on your chest and arms.

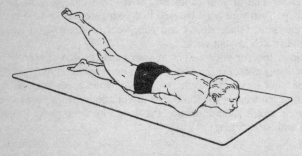

Slowly lower your leg as you exhale. Allow the muscles of your body to relax for a moment. Now, repeat this stretch with your left leg. Then do one more stretch with each leg. Hold each stretch only for as long as it feels comfortable (but no longer than one minute). Take a few moments after each stretch to make sure your body is nicely relaxed.

After practicing these stretches for at least a few days, you can add the following variation: Inhale as you stiffen and raise both legs together, without bending your knees. (You will not be able to raise both legs as high as you could raise only one.)

Continue breathing slowly and deeply. At your own pace, exhale as you slowly lower both legs to the ground.

Turn your head to the side, roll over onto your back, and relax in the Resting Position.

FORWARD STRETCH (NUMBER ONE)

Lie on your back in the Resting Position. Take a moment to become aware of your neck and back muscles.

Now, come to a sitting position and gently hug your knees to your chest. Feel a nice stretch in your lower back. Extend your left leg straight out in front of you. Tuck your right foot into (but not under) the inner side of your left thigh. Reach over your head, lock your thumbs, and inhale deeply; then exhale slowly as you bend forward, keeping your head between your arms and your left leg straight.

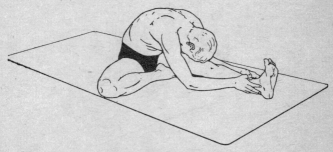

Grasp whatever part of the outstretched leg you can reach—it does not matter whether it is your thigh, knee, or ankle. How far you can stretch is not important. Be sure that your neck is relaxed and that you are feeling a gentle stretch in your neck, back, and the backs of your legs (hamstrings). Breathe normally during this stretch.

As you exhale, let the weight of your body pull you forward. Also, you can gently pull yourself forward with your hands. Remember that bouncing will interfere with your ability to stretch.

If your stretch is gentle but consistent, then you will benefit most. Once your body realizes that you are not going to injure it, it will allow you to relax further into the stretch with each exhalation.

Continue breathing. In this position, it is best not to hold your breath. Try to make each exhalation twice as long as each inhalation—breathing out is the breath of relaxation, as when we say, "Whew!" in a sigh of relief.

When you are finished, lock your thumbs and inhale as you come back up to a seated position. When you get to the top, release your hands and hug your knees to your chest again.

Now extend your right leg. Tuck your left foot into the inner thigh of your right leg. Reach over your head, lock your thumbs, inhale deeply, then exhale slowly as you bend forward, keeping your head between your arms and your right leg straight. Continue the same process that you did on the other side.

When you are through, lock your thumbs and inhale as you come back up. As before, release your hands when you get to the top and hug your knees to your chest again.

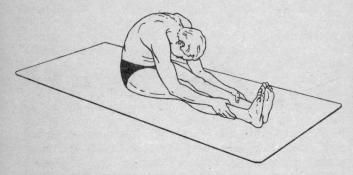

Now extend both legs in front of you. Reach over your head, lock your thumbs, inhale deeply, and exhale slowly as you come forward over both legs. (Remember—how far you can stretch is not important. Most people are not able to stretch as far over both legs as they could over one of them, so be careful not to overdo it.)

Continue breathing. Allow each exhalation to be longer than the inhalation. As you exhale, allow the weight of your body to pull you forward. Remember that bouncing will interfere with your ability to stretch. Be sure that your neck is relaxed.

When you are through, lock your thumbs and inhale as you come back up to a seated position. This time, slowly lower yourself all the way back to the ground. When you have done this, release your hands and bring them back to your sides, assuming the Resting Position on your back. Take a few moments to review your body and notice the effects of the stretching.

SHOULDER STAND

Elevating your legs, as you do during the Shoulder Stand, has many benefits. Among these, it increases the return of blood and lymph from your legs.

The lymphatic system is the sewage system of your body. It carries such things as dead cells and other waste products, and it transports various substances, including fats. The lymph drains into a large vein located near your collarbone. From there, the waste products are pumped through your bloodstream to your liver and kidneys where they are cleared and metabolized.

Unlike blood, which is pumped by your heart, the lymphatic system does not have its own pump. Instead, the lymph is squeezed through the body when your skeletal muscles contract. For example, when you walk, the muscles of your legs contract and squeeze the lymph out of your legs. Unfortunately, since most of us lead rather sedentary lives, the flow of lymph is often sluggish.

The same is true for your blood. Although blood is pumped by the heart, its return from the legs is also stimulated by the contraction of the skeletal muscles. When these muscles are not used, blood—like lymph—tends to pool in the legs. (For many years, the guards at Buckingham Palace and the U.S. Marines have been required to stand for long periods of time without moving. Because of this, blood tended to pool in their legs, so not enough went to their brains—sometimes even causing them to pass out. To prevent this, they now bounce up and down on their toes from time to time. This causes their leg muscles to contract enough to keep the flow of blood moving.)

Elevating your legs allows gravity to help increase the circulation of both lymph and blood. This may help to increase the clearance of waste products from your body.

This Shoulder Stand should not be attempted until you are

quite comfortable with the stretches that you have done so far. Also, you should be able to do the following without difficulty:

Lie on your back in the Resting Position. Bring your feet together. Inhale. Hold your breath for just a moment as you raise your legs about two feet off the ground, keeping them straight. If you are not able to hold them in this position for at least four to five seconds without straining, you should not yet attempt the Shoulder Stand. Also, if you have uncontrolled high blood pressure, shortness of breath, difficulty breathing when you lie flat, congestive heart failure, or a history of problems with your heart, back, head, neck, lungs, or eyes, then you should not do this stretch unless given specific clearance by your physician to do so.

Easy Version. Lie on your back with your legs out-stretched and rest your feet against a wall.

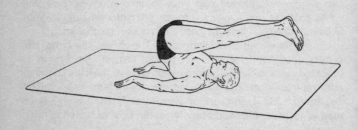

Regular Version. From the Resting Position (on your back), bring your feet together, your arms at your sides, and turn your palms face down. Inhale. While pushing down on your arms and hands for support, bend your knees a little and lift both legs over your head until the knees are over your face. You should be balanced and in control at every point along the way—you are not simply throwing your legs up in the air. Rest here for a moment.

Transfer your hands to the small of your back. Shift your weight to your elbows as you slowly straighten out your body as much as you can. Keep the elbows close to your sides. Breathe normally while maintaining this position.

Stay in this position for only as long as you feel comfortable— but do not overdo it—no longer than a minute or two. If you feel like sneezing, coughing, swallowing, or yawning, come down first before doing so.

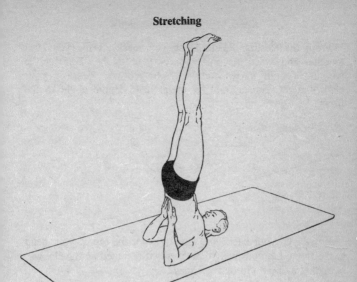

To come down, gently lower your legs over your head, thereby shifting your weight off your elbows. Put your arms back on the floor behind you (where they were). As you exhale, bend your knees and slowly lower your torso and legs as you transfer your weight to your arms for support. When you have lowered yourself completely, return to the Resting Position on your back.

CHEST EXTENSION

This position is the counterpart of the Shoulder Stand, since it stretches you in the opposite direction.

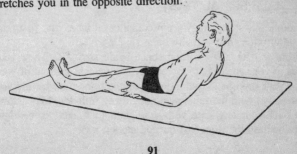

From the Resting Position (on your back), bring your feet together and grasp the underside of your thighs. Transfer the weight of your upper body to your elbows. Keeping your back straight, inhale, and sit up at a 45-degree angle to the floor.

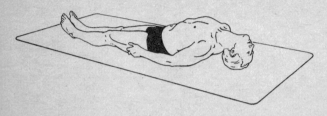

Now, arch your back, and slowly lower the top of your head to the floor. Let your weight be evenly distributed on the elbows, buttocks, and the top of your head.

Continue breathing—take advantage of the extra space that you now have in your thorax and breathe deeply through your nose, filling your chest with air. As before, if you have to swallow, sneeze, cough, or yawn, come out of the position first.

As always, maintain this stretch for only as long as you feel comfortable, but no longer than a minute. When you are ready to come down, transfer your weight back to your elbows, raise your torso off the ground, straighten it out, and then slowly lower yourself back to the ground. Resume the Resting Position on your back.

THE HALF SPINAL TWIST

Although this stretch may seem complicated when you first read the description, it is actually quite simple to do.

From the Resting Position, once again sit up and hug your knees to your chest. Extend your left leg straight in front of you. Place your right hand (palm down) on the floor close behind you for support, with the fingers pointing away from the body. Now, step over your left knee with your right foot, putting the right heel down on the floor just outside the left knee.

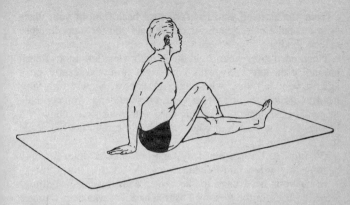

Straighten your left arm and swing it to the right, across your chest. Leaning forward slightly, press the back of your left arm against your right knee, pushing that knee and leg to the left. As you do this, slowly turn your head to the right and look over your right shoulder as you continue to gently push against your right knee with your left elbow. Feel the stretch in your spine. As always, be careful not to overdo it.

Continue to breathe normally. Hold this position for only as long as you feel comfortable, but no longer than a minute or so. Bring your head back to the center and unwind everything.

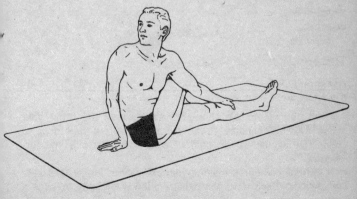

This time, extend your right leg straight in front of you. Place your left hand on the floor directly behind you for support, close to your body.

Now, step over your right knee with your left foot. Reach around your left knee with your right arm and gently push against your left knee with your right elbow. Slowly turn your head to the left and look over your left shoulder as you continue to gently push against your left knee with your right elbow. As before, feel the stretch in your spine, being careful not to overdo it.

Continue to breathe normally, and hold this position for only as long as you feel comfortable.

Bring your head back to the center and unwind everything. Now, lie back in the Resting Position and feel whatever changes have occurred.

FORWARD STRETCH (NUMBER TWO)

From the Resting Position, sit up and cross your legs, campfire style. Reach behind you and take hold of one wrist with your other hand. While sitting up straight, inhale fully, feeling the air as it enters your lungs.

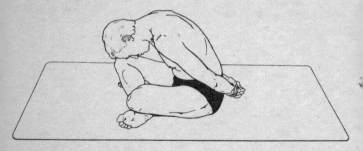

Now, slowly exhale through your nose as you bring your torso forward, bending from your waist. Allow your neck to relax, letting the weight of your head and body pull you forward.

Continue breathing, making your exhalations longer than your inhalations. Each time you exhale, allow your body to relax a little more. Remember not to bounce. If you feel you are going too far, simply pull on your wrist and ease back up slightly. Remember that you are allowing gravity to stretch your body rather than forcing it down.

Continue stretching for as long as you feel comfortable, up to one minute. You may feel a release of tension in your back. When you are finished, sit up slowly and return to the Resting Position on your back. Notice the changes that have occurred.

8. Progressive Deep Relaxation

"For every action there is an equal and opposite reaction." Paradoxically, the easiest way to get your muscles to relax is by first contracting them vigorously.

Progressive Deep Relaxation is a simple yet powerful technique based in part on this phenomenon. It is a sequence of tensing and relaxing the various muscle groups of your body, from your feet to your head.

Your body cannot be relaxed if your mind is agitated. Remember a time when you had difficulty falling asleep. Perhaps you were worrying about things you had to do, things you forgot to do, an argument you may have had, things that you were concerned might happen—so many different thoughts may have run through your mind. Even though the room may have been quiet and your body motionless, you felt quite restless.

To fully relax, therefore, it is not sufficient merely to relax your body—your mind also must be tranquil. To quiet your mind, simply direct your thoughts away from those that are disturbing and toward those that are more peaceful. Of course, this is not always easy to do.

Anxiety, guilt, and fear exist primarily when you think about the past and the future. In Progressive Deep Relaxation, you direct your thoughts to the *present*—by focusing your awareness either on your breathing or on the muscle groups that you will be tensing and relaxing. Focusing in this way is a key to feeling peaceful, because it keeps your awareness in the present moment.

(Moreover, focusing your awareness helps you to experience where you are holding tension so that you can let it go.)

Thus, this is not just a physical exercise—it is a form of meditation. Meditation simply means focusing your awareness.

Just as your state of mind affects your body, the reverse is also true. Relaxing your body helps to relax your mind. That is, the body affects the mind which affects the body which affects the mind . . . and so on. During Progressive Deep Relaxation, you can relax both.

One patient described Progressive Deep Relaxation in this way: "It's great to be totally and completely relaxed—I'd never experienced this before. Even though I'm 'letting go,' I feel like I have more control over my body instead of less."

In this technique, you first bring your awareness to a part of your body. Then, inhale as you stiffen and raise this part no more than an inch off the ground. Then hold your breath as you vigorously contract (squeeze) the muscles in that part of your body for a few seconds. At the signal, "Release!" suddenly relax these muscles and allow that part to drop to the ground—like a dead weight—while allowing the air to rush out of your mouth.

Now to begin. Lie on your back in the Resting Position. As usual, it is best to keep your eyes closed throughout the Progressive Deep Relaxation, since this helps to keep the awareness focused on what you are doing.

Bring your awareness to your right leg. Move it slowly and gently from side to side, noticing how it feels. Inhale deeply through your nose. While holding your breath, stiffen and raise your right leg no more than an inch off the ground—point your toe and contract all of the muscles in your right leg—hold it there for a few seconds . . . now, release! (Allow your leg to drop to the ground as the air escapes from your mouth.) Resume breathing normally.

Now, slowly roll your right leg from side to side until you find a place where it is perfectly balanced, as if it were no longer connected to your body.

Next, bring your awareness to your left leg. Move it slowly and gently from side to side, noticing how it feels. Inhale deeply through your nose. While holding your breath, stiffen and raise your left leg no more than an inch off the ground—point your toe and contract all of the muscles in your left leg—hold it there for a few seconds . . . now, release! Resume breathing normally.

Slowly roll your left leg from side to side until you find a place where it is perfectly balanced, as if it were no longer connected to your body.

Bring your awareness now to the muscles of your pelvis, including your buttocks. Inhale deeply through your nose. While holding your breath, tighten up all of these muscles, raising your pelvis slightly off the ground. Hold it there for a few seconds . . . now, release! Resume breathing normally.

Next, bring your awareness to your lower abdomen. Take in as much air as you can through your nose and force all of it to your abdominal area, causing it to bloat out. Squeeze your abdominal muscles for a few seconds while holding the air in. All at once, allow the air to rush out of your mouth as you relax your abdominal muscles. Resume breathing normally.

Bring your awareness now to your upper chest. Take in as much air as you can through your nose and force all of it to your upper chest, causing it to expand as much as possible. Squeeze the muscles of your chest for a few seconds while holding the air in. Once again, allow the air to rush out of your mouth as you relax your chest muscles. Resume breathing normally.

Bring your awareness now to your hands. Open them and spread your fingers as far apart as you can. Then, clench your hands into tight fists. Now, open your hands again, spreading your fingers as far apart as you can. Once again, clench your hands into tight fists.

Inhale deeply through your nose while continuing to clench your fists. While holding your breath, also contract the muscles in your forearms and arms as you raise them slightly off the ground. Push your shoulders up toward your ears . . . now, release! Resume breathing normally. Slowly roll your arms from side to side and let them come to rest with the palms up.

Bring your awareness now to your head and neck. Slowly roll your head from side to side, allowing your neck to relax as you do so. Now, bring your head back to the center. Inhale deeply through your nose. Hold your breath for a moment and raise your head no more than one-half inch off the ground while contracting the muscles in your neck . . . hold it there for a few seconds . . . now, release! Breathe normally. Once again, slowly roll your head from side to side until you find the place where it is perfectly balanced.

Now, bring your awareness to the muscles of your face. You may be holding some tension there from all of the expressions that you wanted to make recently—but did not. Allow your lower jaw to become slack and move it slightly from side to side. Keeping your eyes closed, raise your eyebrows, and wrinkle your forehead—making a long face. Then, scrunch up your jaw, eyelids, lips, and the other muscles in your face toward the tip of your nose. Make a long face again: open your jaw, raise your eyebrows, and wrinkle your forehead. Then, scrunch everything up together again. Now, push your face muscles in every direction they will go for a few seconds—and then relax. . . .

Breathe normally. Feel the tension coming off your face like steam off a hot frying pan. Slowly roll your head from side to side, allowing your neck to relax. Now, bring your head back to the center.

Without moving any part of your body, just feel yourself sinking into the ground, letting go of any remaining tension, just letting go. . . .

Remember that you are not forcing out the tension—you are simply allowing it to leave your body. Tension serves no useful function. It is like friction in a machine, nothing more. You do not need it, so just allow it to go.

Some people feel as though they are sinking into the ground, feeling very heavy. Others feel as though they are floating.

You may notice that you are hardly breathing at all—your body is so relaxed that it does not need much air. You may feel as though you are swaying a little back and forth each time you inhale and exhale, even though your body is now quite still.

Keeping your eyes closed, now just observe your breathing for a while, without controlling or analyzing it—just step back and watch it. This tends to quiet the mind and allows you to relax even further.

After this, shift your awareness to the mind. Watch the thoughts come and go, without judging them as good, bad, pleasurable, or painful. Without trying to control or direct them, just observe each thought as it comes into your mind—as if it were a bubble coming in, rising to the top, bursting, soon followed by another bubble coming in . . . over and over again.

Now go a step further. See the bubbles as "thoughts," rather than as "*my* thoughts." Just thoughts, nothing more. Continue this process for a while, then return to observing your breathing.

There are exercises to help you direct your mind where you want it to be. We will explore these in more depth in the next sections.

Enjoy this sense of well-being for as long as you want. Notice how secure and content you feel. As you see, it is easy to let go of tension—and it feels so good.

Keep in mind that this Progressive Deep Relaxation did not *bring* this feeling to you—it was there all along. You have simply reduced the body's tension and the mind's chatter that keep you from feeling this way all the time. Once you realize that this sense of well-being—this sense of ease—is always there until it is disturbed, then whenever you feel tense or stressed the question simply becomes, "How did I allow my inner sense of well-being to become disturbed? How did I allow my 'ease' to become 'dis-eased'?" Progressive Deep Relaxation allows us to experience what it means to feel relaxed not because we got what we thought we needed but rather because (at least temporarily) we stopped disturbing what we already have.

When you are ready, inhale deeply through your nose. Feel the air charging your body with life and health. Continue to breathe deeply and slowly as you begin to move your fingers and toes, hands and feet, arms and legs . . . gradually awakening your body. When you are ready, take a minute or two to slowly stretch out everything before getting up.

It is enjoyable to practice the Progressive Deep Relaxation with one or more friends—for the pleasure of seeing each other's face after finishing.

9. Breathing

"Why should I learn how to breathe? What have I been doing all these years?"

At first, it may seem unnecessary, if not ridiculous, to learn how to breathe. But most of us do not realize breathing's important effects on not only our physical but also our emotional states—especially in how we react to emotional stress.

Breathing is a physiological function over which everyone uses both voluntary and involuntary control. However, we are not usually aware of how we breathe during the day—that is, our breathing is involuntary most of the time.

The respiratory center occupies the most primitive, or fundamental, part of the brain: the brainstem. In people with severe brain damage who are in a coma, the respiratory center will usually function even when most of the rest of the brain does not. Because the involuntary control of breathing is so strong, we usually do not have to consciously think about taking a breath every few seconds. This is very useful most of the time, since it frees our awareness to think about more productive activities.

When your breathing is involuntary, it tends to reflect your state of mind. For example, when you are feeling emotionally stressed, anxious, or worried, you will usually find that your breathing is shallow and rapid. On the other hand, when you are peaceful and relaxed, your breathing is usually slow and full.

Likewise, your internal state is affected by how you breathe. When you are feeling emotionally stressed, you can become more tranquil simply by reminding yourself to breathe more slowly and deeply. Most basketball players know this, so they take a slow, deep breath before each foul shot. In a real sense, breathing is a link between your mind and body.

Most of the time, though, we do not breathe slowly and deeply. A typical breath during the day is only about 500 cubic centimeters of air—about one-half pint. However, a full, voluntary inhalation and exhalation will move eight to ten times this amount of air.

Coronary heart disease is due to a lack of oxygen received by the heart. In coronary heart disease patients, anything that decreases the amount of oxygen available to the heart tends to worsen chest pain. For example, the carbon monoxide in cigarette smoke binds with hemoglobin in the blood and prevents it from carrying oxygen to your heart and other organs. On the other hand, when you breathe deeply, you increase the intake of oxygen. (Since hemoglobin carries only a finite amount of oxygen, however, you can increase your oxygen intake only up to a point.) This is especially beneficial for people who smoke. (Quitting is even better.)

People with coronary heart disease have particularly severe difficulty breathing during episodes of chest pain—they often feel as if they cannot get enough air. One participant said before she entered our study: "When I have chest pain, I have a lot of difficulty breathing. Sometimes I have to put my hands on my legs to support my body so I can get a deep breath, but even then I can't get enough." According to another participant, "I used to put out my hand to see if I could get some air and pull it into my chest." Slow, deep breathing may reduce both the anxiety and the severity of chest pain.

COMPLETE DEEP BREATHING

While there are many different types of breathing techniques, the most simple and basic of these—Complete Deep Breathing—is also among the most powerful and useful.

In order to teach it, Complete Deep Breathing is divided into three phases: abdominal breathing, intercostal (chest) breathing, and clavicular (collarbone) breathing. However, it is done as one continuous flow. Each breath begins by filling your abdominal area, then expanding your chest, and finally by raising your clavicle (collarbone).

It is best to practice Complete Deep Breathing for no more than a few minutes at each session. If at any time you feel dizzy or lightheaded, simply resume normal breathing.

To Begin. Sit in a comfortable position, with your back straight but not stiff. Take a few moments to observe your breathing, without trying to change or control it. If you are sitting in a chair, try not to lean against the back of it. Remember that it is best to breathe through your nose, which filters and warms the air.

Abdominal Breathing. Most of us tend to use only our chest when we breathe. Because of this, the abdomen goes in when we inhale and out when we exhale.

Abdominal breathing causes the opposite to occur: breathing begins in the abdomen rather than in the chest. In other words, the abdomen balloons out during inhalations and goes in during exhalations. Because of this, the lungs have much more room to expand, allowing a larger amount of air to enter.

To begin, place your hands on your abdomen. This will help you to be aware of your abdominal muscles as you breathe. Now, contract your abdominal muscles and exhale through the nose as much air as you can. While exhaling, press in with your hands and feel your abdomen going in.

To inhale, breathe in slowly through your nose. With your hands, feel your abdomen expanding as though it were being filled with air. Try not to expand your chest during this part of the technique—only your abdomen is rising as the lower segments of your lungs fill. This is abdominal breathing. Repeat a few times without straining.

Intercostal (Chest) Breathing. After your next inhalation, allow the air to rise into your chest. Feel your ribcage expand.

Clavicular (Collarbone) Breathing. Now add the third portion. Keep inhaling and feel the air rising in your chest. When it reaches the top of your lungs, you will feel your collarbone begin to rise slightly. (At this point, be careful not to draw your abdomen inward.) Remember not to strain.

Now, you have finished a complete inhalation. You have filled your lungs from the bottom to the top with air.

To exhale, repeat the same process in reverse—that is, from

the top to the bottom. As always, it is more relaxing if you take longer to exhale than to inhale.

First, allow some air to escape from the top of your chest, and feel your collarbone lowering as you do so. Next, continue exhaling as you feel the upper and then the lower parts of your chest contracting. Finally, allow the remaining air to come out from your abdominal area, and your abdominal muscles to push out whatever air remains.

That's all there is to it.

It is best to schedule a few minutes each day to practice Complete Deep Breathing, but you can also do it whenever you have some free time.

The more you practice this, the more effective it will be when you need it. You will find that whenever you are feeling anxious, stressed, or worried, a few minutes of Complete Deep Breathing can help to calm you. It works both to prevent harmful reactions to stress and to help relieve them.

You can use this to transform a situation that is usually frustrating and stressful—for example, waiting for a bus, being caught in rush-hour traffic, standing in line, waiting for a late appointment—to one that is more peaceful and manageable. So the next time you find yourself stuck in a traffic jam behind an endless line of motionless cars, take a few seconds simply to breathe slowly and deeply. You may not get there any faster, but you will arrive feeling more relaxed—and less likely to have chest pain or a heart attack en route.

10. Meditation

"In World War II, I fought with all types of weapons systems—105 mm howitzers, bazookas, you name it. But I've never found anything as powerful as meditation."

—BILL F. (research participant)

Remember a time when you were totally absorbed in what you were doing. Hours may have passed, yet it seemed like only a moment. Remember what a good feeling it was to be completely absorbed in the moment—how acute your perceptions were, how clear your thinking was, and how alive you felt. This is meditation.

Meditation is simply focusing your awareness on something. It can be anything—your breathing, a part of your body, a sound, an activity. Although some people still think of meditation as an unusual activity done by men in turbans who sit in caves while chanting in strange languages, there is really nothing mysterious about it. It is not making your mind "blank," nor is it a form of hypnosis. Meditation can produce a state of profound relaxation—but it is much more than this.

Meditation is not something that you have to learn. You already know how to meditate—but you may not always be doing it in a healthy way.

Whenever any form of energy is concentrated and focused, its power increases. Almost everyone has used a magnifying glass to focus the sun's rays on a piece of paper, burning a hole in it. A laser is nothing more than focused light—it is the same type of energy emitted by a light bulb, but because it is focused and coherent, it has the power to burn through steel.

The same may be true of the mind, which is also a form of energy. As with all energy, it seems that awareness may be concentrated and focused. Even our terminology reflects this understanding. For example, we say, "I have been concentrating on this problem all day and now I am able to solve it.'' But the power of the mind goes beyond this.

Whenever you focus your awareness, its effect on your body increases—for better or for worse. The longer you can keep your awareness focused—that is, the longer you are meditating—the greater its effect on your body.

When you are angry or afraid, you are concentrating your awareness very well—that is, your mind is not wandering—but you are meditating on your anger and fear. Since you are concentrating so well, your mind has a profound effect on your body—but it may be a harmful one. As discussed earlier, when you are angry, worried, or afraid, your blood pressure and heart rate may increase dramatically, your arteries are more likely to go into spasm, and your platelets tend to clump together and clog up your blood vessels.

Fortunately, there is a bright side to this: the mind may have a direct positive effect on the body. You can learn to direct your awareness away from harmful meditations and toward beneficial ones—this may provide a double benefit. Also, the more you focus your awareness, the more information you have about what is going on in your body and mind.

Therefore, the question is not, ''Should I learn to meditate?''—because you are already doing so—but rather, ''How can I meditate in a healthy way?''

While the use of meditation in treating coronary heart disease is only beginning to be examined, a variety of investigators have documented its effectiveness in treating related problems, especially hypertension (high blood pressure). A leading researcher in this area has been Herbert Benson, M.D., an associate professor of medicine at the Harvard Medical School and the director of the Hypertension and Behavioral Medicine sections of the Beth Israel Hospital in Boston. He has documented in numerous well-designed studies that regular meditation can reduce blood pressure significantly in many people with hypertension.

Dr. Benson also found that meditation produces a relaxed state—the opposite of the ''fight-or-flight response''—which he has termed the ''relaxation response.'' This response is probably due to several factors, including decreased activity in the sympathetic nervous system (as explained in Chapter 4).

The physiological effects of the profound relaxation produced by meditation are beneficial to people with coronary heart disease. As discussed earlier, angina is the result of an insufficient supply of oxygen to meet the heart's oxygen consumption. Dr. Benson documented that meditation reduces heart rate and the oxygen requirements of the body. In people who meditate, the oxygen consumption decreases 10 to 20 percent; this decrease begins during the first three minutes of meditation. This is an effect produced by propranolol (Inderal), yet without its side effects. (During sleep, oxygen consumption decreases only about 8 percent, and it takes more than four or five hours for this to occur.)

He found additional evidence for the profound relaxation produced by meditation. The brain produces different types of electrical patterns, or waves, which can be measured by an instrument called an electroencephalograph, or EEG. One type, termed "alpha," is present in increased numbers when people feel relaxed. Dr. Benson found that alpha waves increase in intensity and frequency during meditation and are accompanied by a decrease in muscular tension.

He further demonstrated that meditation decreases the frequency of irregular heartbeats (arrhythmias). It is normal for most people to have an occasional "skipped beat," but this can be a serious matter in patients with coronary heart disease. Some types of irregular heartbeats are harmless, but other types may lead to sudden death due to ventricular fibrillation: the heart beats so irregularly and chaotically that it no longer pumps blood effectively. Therefore, since meditation may reduce the frequency of irregular heartbeats, it may reduce the frequency of sudden death due to ventricular fibrillation (although this has not yet been proven).

Dr. Lown is a leading authority on the causes and treatments of irregular heartbeats. At the Brigham and Women's Hospital and the Harvard School of Public Health, his associate, Regis A. DeSilva, M.D., teaches meditation to many patients with life-threatening irregular heartbeats as a supplement to conventional medical therapies.

They have found that about 30 percent of these patients are able to decrease the frequency of irregular heartbeats—sometimes dramatically. Two of three patients who had ventricular tachycardia were able to learn to establish a regular heart rhythm after only three minutes of meditation. This is particularly important because ventricular tachycardia is sometimes a forerunner of sudden death due to ventricular fibrillation. Most patients with life-threatening irregular heartbeats still require drugs and/or surgery.

In more recent studies, Dr. Benson and his associate, Dr. Ruanne K. Peters, found that meditation is helpful in leading a productive life in a large corporation. They randomly divided a group of 120 employees into three groups: one group was taught to meditate one or two times daily (as a "relaxation break"); a second group simply sat quietly for a few minutes without meditating; the third group went through their day as usual. They found that the group which meditated regularly "had lower blood pressures, fewer 'illness days,' and enhanced work performance when compared with the participants in the other groups. They also had fewer symptoms associated with anxiety, including headache, nausea, rashes, diarrhea, mouth sores, difficulty getting to sleep, worrying, and nervous habits such as chewing pencils and biting fingernails."

Meditation brings our awareness into the present moment. Most emotional stress exists when our awareness is in the past or the future—which is where it is most of the time. "I shouldn't have done that"; "I hope things turn out the way I want them to"; "I wish that hadn't happened"; and so on.

Of course, sometimes the present can be quite stressful. One of the most important benefits of regular meditation is that it allows you to better maintain your equilibrium under stressful situations. It is not just that you are able to cope with stress better—situations simply do not bother you as much. Your well-being and equilibrium become less easily disturbed—not just while meditating, but most of the time.

For example, shortly after beginning the program, a dentist in our pilot study was the victim of a theft: his car was broken into and more than five thousand dollars' worth of dental gold was stolen. "Normally, everything about the incident would have caused me pain—from the robbery itself to seeing my car messed up with the black fingerprint powder the police officers used. But I had no pain at all. I took it all in stride—I even kidded the officers about it, went out and got a paper towel and told them to clean it up.

"After my heart attack years ago, things bothered me more than ever. Since learning to meditate, though, things don't bother me nearly as much as they did. I don't know why I used to get so upset before, and I don't know why I don't get bothered as much now."

Meditation helps shift our attention from looking only at the goal (future) to the process of what we are doing now (present). Events are usually less stressful and more enjoyable when we focus on the process rather than on just the goal.

What is the process? It is simply being aware of and enjoying each moment. Life is a process, not just a series of goals to be achieved.

One trait shared by many coronary heart disease patients is a strong sense of goal-oriented behavior and competition. This can interfere with enjoying the process of what is happening.

This does not mean that we should not enjoy our accomplishments. But if we believe that reaching goals is enough to bring us a lasting sense of well-being, then we are setting ourselves up to be disappointed (as described in Chapter 5).

Paradoxically, we can usually achieve even more when we are focused on the process rather than just the goal, because we are thinking more clearly and with less of the anxiety and fear that often accompanies being goal-oriented. And we are able to enjoy what we are doing so much more.

Ted G., one of the research participants quoted in Chapter 5, put it this way a few weeks after the study began: "In my life, I was always waiting for the 'real thing' to start—for the curtain to rise and something better to open up. I'm beginning to realize that life is what happens to you while you're waiting for something else. I still enjoy achieving my goals, but at least I've started looking at the roses along the way. If I can remind myself to stop sometimes and smell them, I'll be even better off."

You can extend this approach to include most things in your life. Whatever you are doing, you will do it better and you will enjoy it more when your awareness is focused on it. In this sense, everything can become a meditation.

For example, I became a little anxious the first time I delivered a baby while a medical student—I learned obstetrics at a high-volume hospital whose philosophy of education was, "Watch one, do one, teach one." I began to think, "What if I make a mistake? What if some rare complication occurs that I can't handle?" I even began to worry that I might drop the baby. (They looked so slippery!) All of these fears and anxieties were based on what might happen—the future—rather than what was happening at that time. When I shifted my awareness to focus on the present, I became less anxious and more aware of the mother's needs, so I was able to better perform the tasks at hand. This helped to transform a somewhat terrifying experience into an enjoyable one.

Even mundane daily tasks—washing dishes, chopping vegetables, and so on—can become a meditation when attention is focused on what is being done. For example, when eating, you will be eating—and because your awareness is on what you are doing and not on business or a magazine or whatever, you will enjoy your food much more and you will be less likely to overeat, because you are aware of how hungry or how full you are.

In this context, meditation does not have a goal. It is both the process and the goal, both the means and the end. If you meditate only to reduce your heart disease or to lower your blood pressure or to "improve your mind," you are thinking about the future instead of meditating, which occurs in the present. Therefore, the best reason for meditating is not that it is "good for you" —although it is—and not that it will help you to live longer— although it may—but simply that it helps you to enjoy the present moment.

MEDITATION: HOW TO BEGIN

1. It is easiest to meditate when your body is relaxed. So, one of the best times to meditate is after finishing the stretching, Progressive Deep Relaxation, and the breathing techniques. If you do not have time to do all of these, then at least a few minutes of complete deep breathing will allow you to begin your meditation much more easily.

2. Find a quiet place where you will not be interrupted. It is helpful to take the phone off the hook, put a Do Not Disturb sign on the door, or do whatever else is necessary to avoid being interrupted.

3. Wait a few hours after eating. Meditation increases the blood flow to your brain. Eating increases the blood flow to your digestive system. Choose one or the other.

4. It is best to keep your eyes closed. It is very difficult to meditate with your eyes open—there are too many interesting distractions.

From the time we get up in the morning until we go to sleep at night, our eyes are assaulted with stimuli, so our awareness is usually directed outward. As a result, we tend to become ignorant of what is going on inside our minds and bodies. Meditation can help you to rediscover yourself.

5. Meditate for only as long as you feel comfortable doing so. Forcing yourself to meditate can agitate your mind even further. Instead, imagine your mind as if it were a bright but mischievous student. As a good teacher, you want to be firm, while maintaining a relaxed sense of humor—knowing when to let the reins out and when to pull them in.

Most meditative traditions recommend sitting in meditation at least twice per day, usually once in the morning and again in the evening, and usually for at least twenty minutes per session. This is fine, but it is best to decide for yourself how much you wish to meditate during each day. In general, the more time you are able to spend in meditation without straining, the greater will be the benefits that you experience. (In deep meditation, you tend to lose track of time because you are so absorbed in the present.)

When you are extremely busy, it may be tempting to postpone meditating until later—but it is at these times when meditation is likely to be of most benefit to you. There is almost always time during the day to meditate for at least a few minutes. The resulting increase in your efficiency and your reduced need for sleep will usually compensate for the short time that you spend in meditation.

6. When your attention wanders, simply bring it back. This will happen over and over again, so do not get discouraged—it is part of the meditative process.

7. It is best to sit with your back straight but not stiff. It does not matter very much where you sit—whether in a chair or on the floor—but it is easier to concentrate if your back is straight.

8. It is best to remain as still as possible while you are meditating. However, you may find that this is not very easy to do, especially at first. Just as your mind tends to wander during meditation, your body tends to become restless. If you can, try to ignore these distractions and continue meditating. If you are unable to do this, then take a moment to do whatever you may need—change your position slightly, scratch where you itch, and so on—and resume meditating.

HOW TO MEDITATE

The easiest form of meditation is also one of the most powerful. Several variations are described below. All of them are based on bringing your awareness either to your breathing or to a sound.

Sit in a quiet place, in a comfortable position, with your eyes closed, and your back straight but not stiff. Without trying to control your breathing, simply become aware of it. Feel the air as it comes in and out of your nose. When your mind wanders, and you find yourself thinking about something else, gently but firmly bring your awareness back to just observing your breathing.

To aid in your concentration, you may find that it is helpful to focus your eyes, even though they are closed, on a point in the center of your forehead just above the bridge of your nose. Also, you may find it helpful to imagine that you are inhaling not only air, but also light.

Now you are meditating.

Another form of meditation is based on focusing your awareness on a sound. The most soothing sounds usually begin with an "aaaahhhh," or an "ohhhhh" sound and end with an "nnnnnnn" or an "mmmmmmm." Thus we find meditative words such as "amen," "shalom," "om," "saalaam," and so on. Traditionally, meditation teachers have maintained that sages in deep meditation heard these sounds and taught them to their students. Whether this is true or not, most of the world's religions incorporate one or more of these sounds as part of their meditative rituals.

However, meditation is not necessarily religious. You can meditate on any of these sounds—or you can create your own. If you do, use one that incorporates these sounds. (Most mothers intuitively realize the soothing power of such sounds, so they hum lullabies to their babies.) It is best, though, to choose or create a word that has no intrinsic meaning to avoid becoming distracted by thinking about the meaning of the word.

For example, one of Dr. Benson's most interesting findings is that the word or sound which one uses to meditate is not very important as long as it is neutral. He studied people who meditated by repeating a Sanskrit word (a mantra) as taught in Transcendental Meditation and found that their responses were identical to those who meditated by observing their breathing or by repeating the word "one." It is the process of meditation that seems to produce the beneficial effects.

Whichever sound you choose, it will be most effective if you stick with it for a while. (An analogy frequently used is that it is more productive to dig one deep well than several shallow dry holes.)

If you meditate on a sound, begin by focusing on your breathing for a minute or so, which will help to quiet your mind. After you have done this for a while, then begin to repeat the sound over and over again. It is easiest to learn this technique by repeating the sound aloud in a quiet voice.

The sound is most effective when the final consonant is prolonged. For example, it is more effective to say "aaahhh-mennnnnnnnnnnnnnnnnnnnnnnnnn" than to repeat aaaaaaaaaaaaaaa-aaaaaaaaaaahhhmennn." Also, it is more soothing to use the lower register of your voice.

Imagine the sound beginning in your solar plexus area (just a few inches above your navel), then filling your chest, and from there coming into the back of your throat, and out of your mouth. Feel your entire body resonating with the sound.

You will find the rate and rhythm that is most comfortable for you. In general, most people find that making one complete sound per exhalation is the easiest way to do this. After a while, continue repeating the sound mentally without repeating it verbally.

As with any meditative practice, your awareness will tend to wander. When it does, gently but firmly bring it back to the sound. As you begin to practice, you will be able to maintain your attention for increasing periods of time before your mind wanders.

Many people find that it is easier to focus their attention on a sound than on their breathing. It is more difficult to keep your mind from wandering when you repeat a sound mentally rather than verbally, but there is the advantage of being able to silently meditate anywhere.

The next chapter—Visualization—takes meditation a step further.

11. Visualization

Your body responds to pictures in your mind.

With your eyes closed, imagine your favorite food. Picture it in as much detail as you can. Notice how it appears: its size, shape, and color. Become aware of how it smells. In your imagination, place a bit of it in your mouth, move it around with your tongue, and notice how it feels in your mouth—is it rough or smooth, crunchy or creamy, sticky or slippery? Notice how it tastes—is it sweet, sour, salty, bitter, spicy, or bland? This is visualization: creating a picture in your mind.

Is your mouth salivating now? This is a simple example of the profound effect visualization can have on your body. While the term may be new, visualization—like meditation—is something that you have been doing for a long time.

Visualization is simply directed meditation. Meditation increases your ability to focus your awareness, thus heightening your powers of concentration; visualization applies this increased power to aid in the healing process. To use an analogy, meditation is sharpening a knife; visualization is cutting with it.

Visualization is not wishful thinking—there is nothing magical about it. Neither is it daydreaming or fantasizing, both of which are unfocused and passive. Visualization is different from these—it is active and directed.

Unlike meditation, visualization gives you the power to direct internal processes somewhat. This can cause physiological changes to occur.

The chapter on meditation describes what happens when you

become angry, worried, or afraid: you are concentrating your awareness extremely well—your mind is not wandering—but you are meditating on your anger and fear. Such focused concentration can have a profound effect on your body—but it is a harmful one.

For example, researchers have found that during times of emotional upset, the nerves and muscles in your body will be in a state of high tension and a marked increase in the frequency and amplitude of nerve impulses can be recorded. Also, your blood pressure and heart rate may increase dramatically, your arteries are more likely to go into spasm, and your platelets may tend to clump together and clog up your blood vessels.

Like meditation, visualization may have both healing and harmful effects, depending upon what you mediate or visualize. For example (and I do not recommend doing this), if you visualize a frightening situation, then the potentially harmful internal changes described above tend to occur—even though you are in a safe place and you may not have been in this situation for years. Dr. Louis Sigler, a New York cardiologist, described one of his patients who was forced to witness the murder of seven family members in a Nazi concentration camp. Recollection (visualization) of this horror produced severe cardiac irregularities in the patient's heart—even though the murders had occurred more than thirty years before and in another part of the world.

Likewise, visualizations may be used to create positive changes in your body and mind, beyond just reducing the negative ones. As with meditation, the question is not, "Should I learn to visualize?"—because you are already doing so—but rather, "How can I visualize in a healthy and productive way?"

Athletes, of course, are interested in anything that improves their mind/body coordination. Some of the most successful athletes have found visualization to be very useful. For example, golf professional Jack Nicklaus once wrote:

> I never hit a shot, even in practice, without having a very sharp, in-focus picture of it in my head. It's like a color movie. First I "see" the ball where I want it to finish. . . . Then the scene quickly changes and I "see" the ball going there. . . . Then there's a sort of fade-out, and the next scene shows me the kind of swing that will turn the previous images into reality.

Visualization

We included visualizations as part of our research program because earlier studies by other investigators indicated that it could be beneficial in treating related problems. However, the use of visualization to treat coronary heart disease had never been studied, so its use is controversial.

As early as 1930, Dr. Edmund Jacobson (a pioneering researcher in this area) documented that visualization can produce measurable changes in the body. For example, he found that when subjects visualized lifting a weight with their right arm, the muscles they would have used to do this contracted a small but measurable amount, even though the arm was motionless. Furthermore, he found that visualization was specific: only the areas that a subject visualized were affected. No changes were detected in the subject's left arm or in other parts of his body.

While Dr. Jacobson's findings were very interesting, they were not very surprising, since he only studied the effects of visualization on the muscles over which we have voluntary control. However, newer studies have shown that visualization can produce changes in systems of the body that scientists once believed were not under voluntary control. In the past ten years, many researchers have documented that almost anyone can learn to control "involuntary" functions such as heart rate, blood pressure, and blood flow to various parts of the body.

Several scientists have investigated the ability to redirect blood flow. In most of these studies, a temperature-sensing electrode was attached to each hand of a subject, who was asked, for example, to close his eyes and visualize that his right hand was on a hot stove and that his left hand was immersed in a bucket of ice water.

The investigators found that the temperature of the subject's right hand increased significantly while that of his left hand decreased. The more blood flow the hands receive, the warmer they become. Therefore, this change in temperature indicated that the blood flow to the right hand had increased—causing the temperature of the right hand to rise—while the blood flow to the left hand decreased, causing its temperature to fall.

Even though the subject was not visualizing the blood flow to his hand, he was able to influence it. Simply by imagining that one hand was very cold and that the other was very hot, the subject was able to influence the underlying mechanisms that caused these physiological changes.

How did this occur? When you visualize changes in your body, these tend to occur even though you may not know the underlying mechanisms required to produce them. In other words, you do not have to know how your nervous system works to be able to harness it effectively. All that is important is to visualize the desired results—*what* you want to happen—not necessarily *how* it happens. To some extent, you can then make this occur.

But why should you care about changing blood flow to your hands?

As described earlier, coronary heart disease is caused by reduced blood flow to the heart. The mechanisms that control blood flow to your hands also may affect the arteries that supply blood flow to your heart: predominantly the ability of your nervous system to constrict and dilate your peripheral and your coronary arteries (via the alpha-adrenergic mechanism described in Chapter 4).

In planning our studies, we reasoned that if visualization could enable a person to influence blood flow to the hands, then perhaps it would enable a patient to increase the blood flow to his heart. While we did not study the effectiveness of any single aspect of our program separately from the others, it is possible that visualization was responsible for some of the measured improvements. As with all components of the program, some people probably responded more to visualization than to other parts of the program.

It is easy to visualize changes in our hands. We are familiar with them—we can see them, we can feel whether they are warm or cold—but the heart is more of a mystery. Therefore, to aid patients in visualizing the desired result—increased blood flow to the heart—we gave each one a diagram of his heart.

These pictures, based on previous diagnostic testing, showed the exact location and extent of the fixed blockages in their coronary arteries. Since these diagrams were pictures, not movies, they could not show the reduction in coronary blood flow caused by active mechanisms such as coronary artery spasm and platelet clumping (described in Chapter 4). However, visualization can. You can "see" a movie in your mind that includes improvement via all of the known mechanisms that cause coronary heart disease, not just the fixed blockages.

The next section will show you how to visualize in a healthy way.

HOW TO VISUALIZE

Visualization is creating a picture in your mind. It is easiest to do after meditating, because meditation helps to focus your awareness. The same eight points that were described in the meditation chapter (pages 110–12) apply equally to visualization.

Many people find that visualization is an easy and natural process. If this is true for you, you may wish to skip the following exercises and begin on page 120.

Visualization is a skill that can be developed. As with any other new skill, your ability to visualize clearly will increase the more you practice. Below are some exercises to help you improve your ability to visualize. Each adds another aspect to the visualization process. Before trying to visualize changes occurring in your heart, it is often easier to begin by visualizing a simple figure.

To begin, draw a circle on a blank sheet of paper. Look at it for a minute or so until you are very familiar with it. Then, close your eyes and continue to "see" the circle in your mind.

Now open your eyes. You may find that the image you saw with your eyes closed is not as sharply focused as the one that you drew. This is normal. Some people who are learning to visualize report that their images seem more like thoughts and ideas than actual pictures. This does not matter—there is no "correct" or "incorrect" way to visualize.

Next, shade the inside of the circle. As before, look at it for a minute or so until you are very familiar with it. Then, close your eyes and continue to "see" the picture in your mind.

Now, without opening your eyes imagine that the color is changing to a different one. For example, if you used a red pen, visualize that the area you colored red is turning to green.

If you have difficulty doing this, open your eyes. Using a different-colored pen or pencil, make a second drawing which is identical to the first except for the color. Now look from the first drawing to the second, close your eyes, and imagine doing the same thing in your mind, "watching" the color change.

Open your eyes.

More information regarding these and other visualization techniques can be found in a book by Mike Samuels, M.D., and Nancy Samuels, *Seeing with the Mind's Eye*.

The next section will show you how to apply these skills to visualize improvements occurring in your heart. This section is designed for people who have coronary heart disease. For people who do not have known coronary heart disease, turn to page 123 to learn how to use visualization as a possible way to help prevent it from occurring.

Some people may find that visualizing the heart provokes anxiety. While I have never encountered this reaction in anyone, if it should occur simply discontinue the visualization and resume meditating on your breathing.

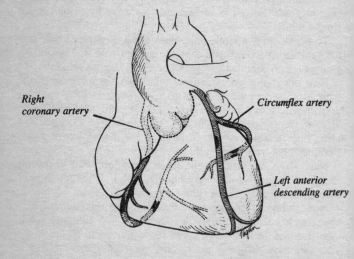

Right
coronary artery

Circumflex artery

Left anterior
descending artery

VISUALIZATION FOR TREATING CORONARY HEART DISEASE

On pages 120–21 are two illustrations of the heart. A heart with severely blocked coronary arteries is on the left. On the right is the same heart, but without any traces of disease.

If you have had prior coronary arteriography (cardiac catheterization), you can ask your physician for the results of your test and substitute a picture of your heart for the one on the left.

Visualization works best when you can imagine your heart beating in three dimensions rather than as a static two-dimensional drawing. Movies of the heart beating are usually available from the public library or from your local chapter of the American Heart Association.

If you do not have coronary heart disease, it is possible that visualization may help to prevent it from occurring, although no one has yet studied this. Begin by examining the illustration on the right, which shows a healthy heart that is free of blockage. Study this closely for a few minutes, skip ahead, and begin reading on page 123. If you have coronary heart disease, continue reading.

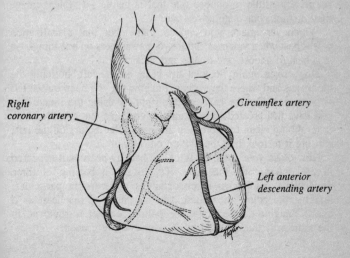

Right coronary artery

Circumflex artery

Left anterior descending artery

Examine the heart on the left. Notice the blockages and how they prevent much of the blood from flowing through the coronary arteries. Spend only a minute looking at this diagram.

Now examine closely the illustration on the right, which shows a healthy heart that is free of blockage. Study this closely for a few minutes. (Spend most of your time looking at the diagram on the right.)

Once again, look at the heart on the left for a few seconds, then quickly move your eyes to the heart on the right, imagining that the heart on the left is becoming like the heart on the right. To do this, create a method of removing the blockages in the coronary arteries. The possible ways of doing this are limited only by your imagination.

In our studies, the patients created a variety of methods. One man imagined a bottle brush swooshing through his coronary arteries and gently cleaning out the blockages. A hardware store owner visualized a Roto-Rooter reaming out the blockages. One man, an artist who works in neon, visualized his coronary arteries as neon tubes with each end hooked up to a power supply that vaporized the blockages. Another person, an oil company worker, imagined an oil derrick drilling through the blockages.

Of course, you may wish to create your own image. If you do so, it is possible to choose one that is gentle—a violent image may disrupt your meditative state.

Whichever image you choose, remember that visualization works best when you concentrate your awareness on one thing—so it is best to choose one image and stick with it.

Now, once again, look at the heart on the left, noticing the blockages and where they occur. Imagine that the heart on the left is becoming like the heart on the right by using the image that you have just created. (For example, visualize that a bottle brush is scrubbing clean the coronary arteries in the picture on the left, causing it to look like the picture on the right.)

Now close your eyes. Imagine the healthy heart as it appeared in the diagram on the right. Try to see it beating in three dimensions, adding as much detail as you can. In particular, imagine the color, the sound, and the shape of the heart as it beats. Imagine the blockages becoming completely removed in the same way that you did when your eyes were open.

*   *   *

Keeping your eyes closed, imagine that your heart is beating strongly and regularly. With each beat, picture the heart pumping efficiently and effortlessly. Visualize that your coronary arteries are relaxed and dilated, allowing blood to flow freely through them. In your mind, see new branches of the coronary arteries growing into areas that need more blood, providing these parts with increased circulation. Continue this for a few minutes.

Repeat this process as often as you wish. If you begin your day this way, your subconscious mind will tend to carry these healthy images throughout your day.

VISUALIZE YOURSELF AS A HEALTHY PERSON

One of the main problems with being labeled a "sick person" is that it tends to create a negative self-image; this may contribute to further illness in a vicious cycle as a self-fulfilling prophecy. As one patient told me, "I feel weak and I am in pain. I can't do the things I want because I feel so bad. My doctor told me that I am a sick person; my friends and family tell me that I'm sick. The more I hear that I'm a sick person, the more I begin to think of myself as one. This makes me feel even more frightened and depressed, which takes away my desire to do anything—making me feel even more stressed."

Visualization can help to break this cycle. Whenever you visualize your heart improving, end the session by seeing yourself as a healthy person. The visualization described below is designed to help extend the possible improvements in your heart to the rest of you.

Begin by thinking of an activity that you used to enjoy but have not done for a while because you have been sick. (Some of the patients in our studies imagined themselves playing tennis or other sports, working in a garden, making love, working, taking long walks, or doing other pleasurable activities.)

Now, while sitting in a comfortable, quiet position, close your eyes and "see" yourself (in your mind) doing this activity. Imagine "seeing" the surroundings through your eyes while you are doing the activity, not as another person would see you. Use all of your senses: visualize motion, color, sound, touch, taste, smell, and so on. The more details you can include, the more effective (and enjoyable) will be your visualization.

Visualize that you are enjoying this activity and that you are completely free of pain while doing it. Imagine yourself as completely healthy, full of energy and life, with all of your organs (including your heart, of course) functioning normally. See yourself as a well person.

Continue doing this for as long as you like. Open your eyes when you have finished. How do you feel?

Of course, just because you have visualized an activity does not mean that you instantly have become well and that you can immediately do this activity. For example, if you have not exercised in a long time, it would be foolish to run out and begin playing five sets of tennis. Your body needs time to begin healing itself. Visualization may help.

THE OPEN HEART VISUALIZATION

This visualization is the most challenging—and perhaps the most powerful—of all the techniques in the program. As one of the patients said on the last day of the study, "This one is tough. If we had learned it in the beginning, it would have been too much for me to accept."

By now, you know the effects of stress on your heart and how it may reduce blood flow via the mechanisms described earlier. We also have discussed how visualization may have harmful as well as healing influences on your body.

One of the most harmful visualizations comes from the anger and resentment that we often hold inside. Anger is not necessarily harmful—if it is expressed and resolved. But when we carry it with us from day to day, we tend to visualize in a way that may be harmful to the heart.

Although scientists are only beginning to explore this area of research, our language reflects this understanding. We speak of an angry, callous person as being "hardhearted" or "closed-hearted" or "coldhearted," whereas we describe one who is loving and happy as being "openhearted" (no blockages in the coronary arteries?) or "warmhearted" (due to increased blood flow?).

At one time or another, all of us have been treated unfairly. We often respond by feeling angry. When this anger is not expressed and resolved in a constructive way, we may internalize it and carry it with us from day to day. Whenever we think about—visualize—the person or situation that caused our anger, we tend to become upset again. After a while, this emotional stress may produce chronic injuries to the walls of the coronary arteries (via the mechanisms described in Chapter 4); in turn, this may lead to coronary heart disease.

Years may pass, but if the anger remains unresolved it may cause harmful effects as powerful as on the day of the original incident. For example, while I was a medical student, a heart patient told me that he was still intensely angry at an army buddy for betraying him to the enemy in World War II. He felt completely justified in his anger—and he probably was. Yet his anger was not hurting the army "buddy" at all, who in fact had been killed years earlier during the war. But it was hurting the patient quite a lot; just telling me the story caused him to have severe chest pains. In effect, the patient was giving away the power to make himself sick or well, and ultimately, to live or die, to the man whom he most despised—someone who had been dead for years.

To one degree or another, most of us do this. But we have a choice: we can take back what we have given away. This does not require other people to change at all. We need only to change our perceptions—how we view them.

In short, we can learn to forgive. We can learn to open our hearts. In this context, to forgive is not a sign of weakness; it is the strongest and healthiest thing we can learn to do.

"Forgiveness" is a concept that is often misunderstood. It need not be viewed as religious or unselfish. We forgive not to be a "good person," not to get a gold star, not to go to heaven—but simply because it is in our self-interest to do so. It's pragmatic: by doing this, we can feel more free of stress, pain, and disease.

Begin by sitting in a comfortable position with your eyes closed. For the next few minutes, direct your awareness to observing your breathing, as described earlier.

Keeping your eyes closed, bring to mind an image of a person with whom you are angry. (Visualize only one person.) Imagine someone who has done something to you that you have never quite been able to forgive. Try to see this person's face in as much detail as you can.

Now, imagine that you are reliving the incident. Remember as many details as you can and include these in your visualization.

Notice how you feel—including the changes in your breathing, heart rate, muscular tension. Since the incident occurred, physical and emotional stress has often resulted whenever you have thought of this person. In this context, you have given to this person the power to produce these unpleasant and potentially harmful changes in you. Your anger is not affecting the other person, but it may be hurting you.

You are not able to change the other person—but you don't need to. Simply by changing the way you view him you will change the way you react and how you feel.

To accomplish this, transform the way that you are visualizing this person. Instead of seeing him as being malicious, evil, or heartless, see him as a small child or as an ignorant adult—one who should know better but does not. If you prefer, choose another image—whatever works to transform your feelings of anger or hatred into those of compassion: "Isn't it sad that he's that way, but I don't have to let it affect me. I can forgive him for what he did—it doesn't matter anymore. It's all in the past—it is only in the present because I'm keeping it here. Once I forgive him, then I'm freer."

Continue this process for a few minutes (or as long as you feel comfortable). If at any time you feel too uncomfortable, simply redirect your awareness to observing your breathing.

After you have completed this process, direct your awareness to observing your breathing. Continue doing this for a few minutes more.

After you feel comfortable with these visualization techniques, then go a step further. Keeping your eyes closed, bring to mind an image of yourself. In particular, imagine an episode in your life that you regret—something that you did or did not do, for which you never have quite forgiven yourself. (You don't have to tell anyone what it is, of course, just visualize it.)

As before, imagine that you are reliving that episode. Remember as many details as you can, and include these in your visualization.

Again, notice how you feel—the changes in your breathing, heart rate, muscular tension, and so on.

Now, transform the way in which you are visualizing yourself. Feel the same compassion for yourself that you extended to the person in the previous visualization. In your mind, hear yourself saying, "I made a mistake and learned from it. I was ignorant— perhaps I should have known better. The past has passed—I have suffered enough. I forgive myself for what happened." If you are sincere, you probably will notice that you feel more relaxed.

After you have completed this process, then observe your breathing. Continue doing this for a few minutes or so, then open your eyes when you are ready.

Anger is not always inappropriate. Sometimes it can be quite healthy to be angry, and it is usually better to express anger than to repress and turn it inward. Meditation and visualization can help to make you more aware, both of your feelings and of those of others. But they also help to put things in perspective. After a few weeks of regular meditation, you may find that you are not as distressed by trivial events that used to be so upsetting. And when you become angry, you can feel it clearly, express it constructively—and let it go. It is when you hold on to anger long after it has served its purpose that it may become destructive.

When you forgive people, it does not absolve them from responsibility for what they have done. It does not excuse them— it simply frees *you* from being affected in a harmful way.

Likewise, forgiving yourself does not absolve you from your responsibilities, but it will help to free you from the pain, stress, and guilt that you may impose on yourself. You will then be able to see more clearly and accomplish whatever needs to be done in a more constructive way.

Very few of us are ready to look honestly at ourselves. Real change may involve a lot of pain. As Harry Stein writes, "We all have within us a thousand ways to avoid unpalatable truths, countless cul-de-sacs of the heart and mind. When we are unloved, it is because others are callous; when we are incapable of love, others are unlovable. We will be glib about our problems, or impervious or maudlin, but almost never will we be utterly straight with ourselves. And that being that, all our efforts to make ourselves happy (the most abused word in the English language) will invariably end up as emotional tap dancing, noisy motion leading absolutely nowhere. The truth is, most of don't know and don't want to know."

It is so much easier to blame others—our parents, our genes, our lovers, our gods—than to acknowledge, in the often-quoted lines of Pogo, "We have met the enemy and he is us." Meditation and visualization can help us to become more aware of who and what we are rather than what we think we "should" be. When we can acknowledge what we feel—the negative as well as the positive—and accept this without flinching or condemning, then we are more free. To acknowledge who we are is the first step in changing for the better. To the degree we can forgive ourselves, then we can forgive others. To the degree we can have this compassion for others—when we truly open our heart—then the barriers that separate us begin to fall away. As the barriers begin to crumble, stress is reduced and healing can begin.

Perhaps all of us can benefit from this type of "open heart" surgery.

12. How to Quit Smoking

"The unfortunate thing about this world is that good habits are so much easier to give up than bad ones."

—SOMERSET MAUGHAM

"The only way to stop smoking is just to stop—no ifs, ands, or butts."

—EDITH ZITTLER

You know it's bad for you. But it's even worse than you think.

Smoking is slow-motion suicide. In 1979, the U.S. Surgeon General published a book, *Smoking and Health,* that summarized the health consequences of smoking. Just this *summary* of the research documenting how smoking contributes to disease (including coronary heart disease) was well over a thousand pages in length.

There are many good reasons to stop smoking, and there are various techniques for doing so. The key to all of them is motivation. There are no magic tricks. You have to decide you want to do it for yourself. When you do decide—quit!

The stress reduction techniques described on the preceding pages—especially the breathing techniques—can help. Instead of reaching for a cigarette when you feel tense, simply take a few slow, deep breaths. The following suggestions are from a pamphlet prepared by the National Cancer Institute, "Clearing the Air":

- List all the reasons why you want to quit. Every night before going to bed, repeat these.
- Decide positively that you want to quit.
- Set a target date for quitting—perhaps a special day like your birthday, your anniversary, or a holiday. If you smoke heavily at work, quit during your vacation. Make the date sacred, and don't let anything change it.
- Bet a friend you can quit on your target date.
- Ask your spouse or a friend to quit with you.

- Reach for a glass of juice instead of a cigarette for a midday lift.
- Think of quitting in terms of one day at a time. Tell yourself you won't smoke today, and don't.
- On the day you quit, throw away all cigarettes and matches. Hide lighters and ashtrays.
- Visit the dentist, and have your teeth cleaned to get rid of tobacco stains.
- Keep very busy on the day you quit. Go to the movies, exercise, take long walks, go bike riding.
- Buy yourself a treat. Do something special to celebrate.
- During the few days after you quit, drink large quantities of water and fruit juice. Try to avoid alcohol, coffee, and other beverages with which you associate cigarette smoking.
- If you miss the sensation of having a cigarette in your hand, play with something else—a pencil, a paper clip, or a marble.
- Get plenty of rest.
- Absorb yourself with activities that are the most meaningful and satisfying to you.
- When you get the "crazies," practice the deep breathing, stretching, meditation, and progressive deep relaxation techniques. If you can't sit long enough to do these, then take a shower.

Within twelve hours after you have your last cigarette, your body will begin to heal itself. The levels of carbon monoxide and nicotine in your system will decline rapidly, and your heart and lungs will begin to repair the damage caused by cigarette smoke.

Within a few days, you will begin to notice some remarkable changes in your body. Your sense of smell and taste will return. Your smoker's hack will be diminished or even gone.

As your body begins to repair itself, you may feel worse before you begin to feel better. The nicotine found in cigarettes is addictive; when you quit, your body goes through withdrawal. You may feel edgy and more short-tempered than usual. These are only temporary and signal that your body is detoxifying itself.

Most important, you will begin to feel really alive—more clearheaded and full of energy. And you will be free from the mess, smell, expense, and dependence of cigarette smoking.

Good luck!

Part Three
THE DIET

13. Introduction to the Diet

It is easy to eat in a healthful way.

This is not a diet in the usual sense—there are no lists of "you can eat this" and "you can't eat that," because dietary requirements vary from person to person and from time to time. And even more than being healthy, most of us want to feel unregimented and free to choose.

Instead, foods are classified into a spectrum of five categories: Group 1 includes foods that, for most of us, seem to be the most nourishing; Group 5 includes those that appear to be the least so. Groups 2 through 4 are intermediate. You decide what plan on this spectrum is best for you. This is only a guide, not a bible.

The participants in our research studies were served foods from Group 1 only. If you have coronary heart disease, you are likely to show the greatest improvement if you limit yourself to foods from this group, with excursions into Groups 2 and 3 from time to time. Likewise, if you wish to reduce your risk of developing coronary heart disease, then you may wish to derive most of your diet from these foods.

It is easiest to begin with whatever you are now eating and work your way toward the Group 1 end of the spectrum. Gradual changes are usually less stressful than abrupt ones. After a while, instead of fighting a daily battle of self-denial, many people find that they simply lose interest in Groups 4 and 5.

The rationale for these food groupings has been detailed throughout this book. A recurrent theme has been that coronary heart disease appears in many ways to be a disease of excess. This seems to be especially true with respect to diet. Most Americans consume excessive amounts of cholesterol, fat, protein, and calories. As stated earlier, the body makes all of the cholesterol it needs. It is the excessive amount in our diet that causes problems.

Cholesterol is found only in foods of animal origin. *There is no cholesterol in fruit, vegetables, grains, beans, or any plant-based food.* While fat is found in almost all foods, it is usually highest in those of animal origin. Also, most animal fat is saturated, while most vegetable fat (except for a few foods, such as coconuts, olives, and avocados) is unsaturated. Saturated fat tends to raise blood levels of cholesterol, while unsaturated fat tends to reduce it.

Part One of this book describes how a diet that is high in animal products (and thus high in saturated fat and cholesterol) may lead to coronary heart disease. A few additional studies are summarized below. It is evidence of this type that forms the basis for the food classification groups of the diet.

There is nothing new about this way of eating; neither I nor anyone else can claim credit for it. Groups 1 and 2 are simply vegetarian—no meat, fowl, or fish. While vegetarian diets have in the past been associated in this country with people who are "a little crazy," including some strange cults or fanatics, most people throughout the world have eaten primarily vegetarian foods until recently. It is still the way that most of the world eats—except for the industrialized countries like ours where coronary heart disease is epidemic.

Coronary heart disease is a twentieth-century phenomenon—and so is the emphasis on animal products in our diet. In the early 1900s, coronary heart disease was a comparatively rare illness. In 1968, the renowned cardiologist Paul Dudley White reviewed the hospital records of eight hundred patients who had been under his care as an intern at the Massachusetts General Hospital in 1912–1913. Only eight of these—1 percent—were diagnosed as having coronary heart disease. Today, the number might be closer to 40 percent or more.

The rise of coronary heart disease in the United States paralleled the changes in U.S. dietary habits. As the consumption of animal fat and cholesterol began to rise during this century, so did the incidence of coronary heart disease.

Introduction to the Diet

People in most of the world—the "underdeveloped countries"—have never increased their consumption of animal products. In these countries, coronary heart disease is still a rare illness. The average cholesterol level in these countries is around 140–160 mg percent. In contrast, the average cholesterol level in Americans is about 210–230 mg percent. Residents of underdeveloped countries who move to the U.S. and adopt the typical American diet have much higher risk for developing coronary heart disease, although residents who move here and maintain their former (plant-based) diet remain at low risk.

A few groups of Americans have maintained their largely vegetarian diets despite increasing modernization. For example, Seventh-Day Adventists are one large group who have done so. In a six-year study of 24,000 vegetarian Seventh-Day Adventist (SDA) men, Dr. R. L. Phillips found that the mortality rate from coronary heart disease was much less in SDA men than in the general population. In SDA men and women age thirty-five to sixty-four, the mortality from coronary heart disease was 72 *percent* less than the general population in the same age group. In those who were at least sixty-five years of age, the mortality from coronary heart disease was only one-half that of the general population.

This decreased risk of coronary heart disease mortality was partially because SDAs do not smoke. To control for this and for other factors that may have been unique to SDAs, the investigators compared meat-eating SDAs with those who consumed no animal products (strict vegetarians). Both groups were nonsmokers, yet the risk of fatal coronary heart disease among the nonvegetarian men (ages thirty-five to sixty-four) was *three times greater* than vegetarian men of comparable age—suggesting that the vegetarian diet may account for a large share of this low risk. Those who were vegetarian but who also consumed milk and egg products had a risk of fatal coronary heart disease that was intermediate between these two groups—about one-third less than the nonvegetarian men.

Two of the largest and perhaps most definitive studies of the role of diet in coronary heart disease have been the Framingham Heart Study and the Seven Countries Study.

The Framingham Study was a twenty-four-year study of the life habits and health of almost six thousand men and women in the small town of Framingham, Massachusetts (just outside of

135

Boston). According to William P. Castelli, M.D., the scientific director of the study:

> Many people (even doctors) feel that if your cholesterol is average you are normal. Too few people realize that an average American cholesterol level (about 210–230 mg%) is a dangerously high level indeed. As we have discovered from studying the natural history of coronary heart disease as it occurs in America and elsewhere in the world, a safe cholesterol level is one around 150–160 mg%. Very few Americans over age 30 (fewer than five per cent) have such a value. Most of the heart attacks in America develop in people whose blood cholesterols are between 230–250 mg%, levels few doctors consider serious enough to treat. Yet when we were teenagers, most of us had a cholesterol around 150–160 mg%. . . . In virtually all instances where reversibility [of coronary heart disease] occurs, the level of cholesterol attained is in the vicinity of 150–160 mg%. Such a level is attainable in humans, without the aid of drugs, practically only in people who have gone largely vegetarian.

The Seven Countries Study was a massive ten-year study of more than twelve thousand men in—not surprisingly—seven countries: the United States, Italy, Greece, the Netherlands, Yugoslavia, Finland, and Japan. The investigators, led by Dr. Ancel Keys, found that diet, blood pressure, and blood levels of cholesterol were strongly related to coronary heart disease. The people of Finland had the highest percentage of saturated animal fats in their diet, the highest cholesterol levels in their blood—and the highest death rate from coronary heart disease. The U.S. death rate was not much less.

However, in countries such as Italy and Greece, where much of the diet is derived from plants (including most of the oils used in cooking), the death rate for coronary heart disease was much lower. In Japan, even more of the diet is plant based (only 10 percent of the diet is fat, compared with 40 to 50 percent in the U.S.)—and the death rate from coronary heart disease was *one-tenth* that of Finland.

In another study, Dr. Richard Shekelle and his colleagues followed nineteen hundred middle-aged men in this country over a twenty-year period. They reported in 1981 that, overall, the more saturated fat and cholesterol in a person's diet, the higher the level of cholesterol in his blood was likely to be. And the higher his cholesterol level, the greater was his risk of early coronary death. Men whose intake of cholesterol and saturated fat was lowest had a coronary death rate that was one-third lower than those whose diets were highest in these.

Because of evidence such as these studies, the U.S. Senate Select Committee on Nutrition and Human Needs issued a report in 1977 that specified dietary goals for all Americans. One of the report's most important recommendations was that Americans reduce their consumption of cholesterol and saturated fat. This historic action (no federal agency had previously endorsed the view that malnutrition might include *overconsumption* of food) was followed by similar statements from the Department of Agriculture, the Surgeon General, and the Department of Health, Education, and Welfare. In 1982, the National Cancer Institute made similar recommendations in hopes of reducing the incidence of certain types of cancer.

And in a recent position paper, the American Dietetic Association, the main professional association of registered dieticians, stated: "a growing body of scientific evidence supports a positive relationship between the consumption of a plant-based diet and the prevention of certain diseases [such as coronary heart disease]. A well planned diet, consisting of a variety of largely unrefined plant foods supplemented with some milk and eggs meets all known nutrient needs. Furthermore, a total plant diet can be planned to be nutritionally adequate, if attention is given to specific nutrients which may be in a less available form or in lower concentration or absent in plant foods."

All foods contain three important constituents: protein, fat, and carbohydrate. Somehow, most of us have been conditioned to think of protein as "good", fat as "bad," and carbohydrate (starch) as, well, "fattening." Let's examine each of these.

PROTEIN

Protein is amazing. It is present in countless forms in the body, from the framework of most structures to the microscopic enzymes that regulate virtually all physiological reactions. Proteins form the antibodies that defend us, regulate the genes that define us, and constitute much of the bones, muscles, and connective tissue that hold us together. It is not surprising, therefore, that most of us want to be sure that we eat enough of it.

Unfortunately, as with almost everything in life, it is possible to get too much of a good thing. There is an almost mystical reverence that most of us have learned to associate with protein, equating "protein" with "good nutrition," and the more the better. The idea that we cannot get enough protein without eating meat is based on a misconception of the nature of food. Protein is contained, at least to some degree, in virtually *all* foods, not just animal products. For most people in this country, the problem is that we eat *too much* protein—at least twice as much as we need.

It is not clear whether too much animal protein is harmful to the heart, although there are some studies by Dr. K. K. Carroll and others to suggest that it may be (see Chapter 4). Excessive protein is stored (as fat) or excreted. For this reason, too much protein may be harmful to people with kidney or liver disease (the organs of excretion). Also, there is some evidence to suggest that excessive protein may promote the loss of calcium, and this may lead to bone demineralization.

Protein is formed from building blocks, called amino acids. Like fats and carbohydrates, each amino acid contains carbon, hydrogen, and oxygen. Amino acids also contain nitrogen, and this allows the amino acids to link together in long chains, cross-linked like a ladder every so often for stability. The sequence of amino acids determines the type of protein and what it can do. Just as the twenty-six letters of the English alphabet can form an endless number of words, there are twenty-two different kinds of amino acids in the body; these amino acids can combine to form countless varieties of proteins.

Thirteen of these amino acids can be manufactured by the body (the "nonessential amino acids"). Nine of these—the "essential amino acids"—cannot, and they must be supplied in the diet each day. Although all of these nine amino acids are equally essential, only three—lysine, tryptophan, and methionine—are critical in most diets, since the others are more plentiful in most foods.

All of the essential amino acids can be supplied in a well-

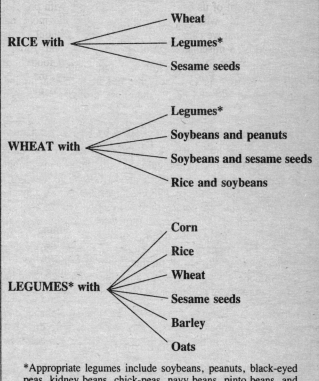

If you combine vegetable proteins in the same meal in any of the ways suggested below, you will obtain complete protein equivalent to the protein in meat and other animal foods.

RICE with
- Wheat
- Legumes*
- Sesame seeds

WHEAT with
- Legumes*
- Soybeans and peanuts
- Soybeans and sesame seeds
- Rice and soybeans

LEGUMES* with
- Corn
- Rice
- Wheat
- Sesame seeds
- Barley
- Oats

*Appropriate legumes include soybeans, peanuts, black-eyed peas, kidney beans, chick-peas, navy beans, pinto beans, and lima beans.

balanced vegetarian diet. The protein contained in plant foods provides the same animo acids as that contained in animal foods. The idea that animal products provide a special kind of protein is a myth. By eating a varied, plant-based diet, you can obtain all of the protein that you need without consuming the excessive fat and cholesterol that may lead to coronary heart disease.

However, no single plant source contains all of the essential amino acids in sufficient quantity. Fortunately, one type of food may be high in one amino acid and low in another, while a different food may have the opposite proportions. By combining two or more different foods at the same meal (some studies suggest that during the same day is sufficient), you can obtain all of the essential amino acids.

For example, beans are high in lysine and tryptophan but low in methionine. Rice is low in lysine but high in methionine. Eating a meal of rice and beans, therefore, provides a complete protein.

Each category of food—legumes (beans and peas), grains, vegetables, and fruits—tends to share the same strengths and deficiencies of amino acids. So, it is not necessary to carry around complicated food tables, calorie charts, or protein-combining formulas each time you have a meal. *As long as you eat a variety of whole foods from each food category during the day and an adequate amount of calories, then you can be assured that you are obtaining all of the high-quality protein that you need*—no different than the quality of protein found in steak. (This is not always true for pregnant women, children, and postsurgical or burn patients whose protein requirements are increased.)

Of importance is what you *don't* get along with the steak: the excessive saturated fat and cholesterol that may lead to coronary heart disease.

FAT

Fat is not "bad"; we simply eat too much of it. For most Americans, fat supplies more than 40 percent of the dietary calories. Yet very little dietary fat is required.

The only fat required in the diet is a substance called linoleic acid, found in almost any polyunsaturated vegetable oil (safflower, soy, corn, sesame, and cottonseed oils are particularly high in this). Only a tablespoon per day is enough, including what is already supplied in the diet. Beyond this, for most people, the less fat you eat, the better. Like protein, most of us tend to eat too much fat. Saturated fats—animal fats—are not required in the diet at all. Your body can synthesize whatever fat you need from protein and carbohydrate.

The major role of fat is to store energy. Nine calories of energy can be stored per gram of fat. Proteins and carbohydrates can store only four calories of energy per gram. This is a double-edged sword: while this makes fat a very efficient storehouse of energy, it also means that it is easy to eat an excessive amount of calories when the proportion of fat in the diet is high. Also, a large amount of energy expenditure is required to "burn off" the excessive fat that most people eat. Fat also helps to cushion internal organs, to store fat-soluble vitamins (A, D, E, and K), and to reduce the loss of body heat during cold weather.

If we currently eat too much fat and too much protein, what should we be eating?

CARBOHYDRATES

Complex carbohydrates—starch—form the basis of the diet in Groups 1 and 2. The carbohydrates in whole foods such as whole wheat, beans, unrefined grains, fruits, and vegetables (complex carbohydrates, in contrast to simple carbohydrates like refined sugar and white flour pastries) are a very efficient source of energy.

While fats and proteins can be metabolized into energy, the body has the easiest time with carbohydrates and the fewest waste products to contend with. Carbohydrates consist of long chains of glucose and similar compounds, and they are easily broken down to glucose, which is the primary fuel of cellular metabolism. This spares the protein for use in building tissues, repairing cells, and so on, instead of "wasting" it for conversion to energy. For this reason, people on a high-carbohydrate diet are using their food more efficiently, and have fewer nitrogen waste products to excrete. When intake of carbohydrates is low, fat is converted to energy less efficiently, and toxic substances known as ketones are produced, placing an additional strain in the liver and kidneys.

The Diet

Unfortunately, most of us have learned to think of carbohydrates as fattening, filling foods that crowd out the "real" nutritious foods. This is simply not true. Carbohydrates have the same number of calories per gram—four—as protein. *Fat* is fattening.

Part of the reason for this misconception is that starches, or complex carbohydrates, have formed a progressively diminished part of the American diet over the past fifty years, while the intake of simple carbohydrates, such as sugar and alcohol, has increased dramatically. Sugar and alcohol provide only empty calories and crowd out more nutritious foods.

There is nothing wrong with small quantities of sugar. If you have ever chewed on sugar cane, or eaten too much honey or too many apples, you know that you can eat only a certain amount before you get a queasy feeling that keeps you from overdoing it. Also, the sheer bulk prevents overeating. Unfortunately, we have refined away the "warning signals" that are present in the natural product, so it becomes possible to eat virtually unlimited quantities of refined sugar. On the average, we now eat more than a pound of sugar every three days. This adds up to a lot of calories—15 to 20 percent of our daily caloric intake—so it is not surprising that carbohydrates are considered fattening.

In the process of refining out the warning signals, the indigestible fiber that slows the absorption of sugar into the bloodstreams has also been removed. When complex carbohydrates are eaten in proper combination at a meal, glucose is gradually absorbed into the bloodstream over a period of several hours, maintaining a fairly even level of blood sugar. However, refined sugar is digested and absorbed very quickly, causing a higher peak and, in many cases, a letdown that soon follows.

Several studies have demonstrated that changing to a high-carbohydrate diet improves exercise tolerance, a fact that has not been lost on athletes. For example, about a third of the Dallas Cowboy football players skip the steak at their pregame meal and choose instead high-energy carbohydrate dishes such as—no kidding—French toast, oatmeal, or toast and honey. Both wide receiver Butch Johnson and tight end Billy Joe DuPree follow a vegetarian meal plan. In training camp, players are advised to keep fat and proteins to a minimum.

Groups 1 and 2 are high in complex carbohydrates. Most people who limit themselves to Groups 1 and 2 find that they can eat until they are satisfied, yet they do not gain weight—in our study, there was an average weight loss of ten pounds in three weeks. If you are obese, a diet that is high in complex carbohydrates may help you to lost weight. Why? Because you are consuming less fat (which has more than twice the calories per gram), you will feel "full," and you will not have the sense of deprivation that you may have felt when dieting—giving you a psychological lift that may help to break the cycle of overeating caused by depression.

VITAMINS AND MINERALS

The richness in minerals and vitamins of plant foods is well known. There are, however, a few exceptions that may be of concern only if animal products are *totally* excluded (which I do not recommend for most people). Vitamin B_{12} is the only nutrient that is difficult to get from a totally plant-based diet, but sufficient quantities can easily be obtained from nonfat yogurt. Vitamin D results by exposure of skin to sunlight. (A sufficiency of both of these can be ensured by a simple multivitamin.)

Calcium and riboflavin are also obtained by eating nonfat yogurt. For the total vegetarian, calcium sources include regular servings of many of the dark green vegetables, such as broccoli, collards, kale, mustard, and turnip greens; legumes; fortified soy milk; and some nuts such as almonds or seeds such as sesame. Dark green leafy vegetables are also good sources of riboflavin.

Iron deficiencies are widespread and not limited to vegetarians. Ascorbic acid increases iron absorption by maintaining iron in a reduced, more soluble form. Iron supplements, especially in menstruating women, are often advisable.

Zinc is found in green leaf vegetables or stem vegetables or in the pulp of fruit. Phytates, which interfere with zinc absorption, are decreased during the yeast fermentation of whole wheat flours during breadmaking.

In summary, the best diet for most people is based on foods that are in the form closest to when they were harvested. This

The Diet

includes fresh fruit, unrefined grains (such as whole wheat bread, oatmeal, brown rice, dried beans), fresh vegetables (steamed corn, baked potato), and so on.

Healthful eating need not be boring, bewildering, or time-consuming. Chapters 14–20 include a detailed description of how to prepare the diet, with innovative recipes by Martha Rose Shulman that are tasty and attractive as well as nutritious.

Five Food Groups

GROUP 1

Grains

All whole grains, including:
barley
bread
buckwheat/buckwheat flour
bulgur
cereals (oatmeal, granola without coconut or sugar, shredded wheat)
corn/popcorn/corn meal/ corn flour/corn grits
crackers (whole wheat, rice)

millet
oats
rice (whole grain, wild)/rice flour
rye/rye flour
sorghum grain
soybeans/soybean flour
tortillas
triticale
wheat (whole grain, cracked, rolled, flour, bran, germ)

Vegetables

All fresh vegetables, such as:
artichokes
asparagus
bamboo shoots
beets
broccoli
Brussels sprouts
cabbage (all types)
carrots
cauliflower
celery
chili peppers

collards
corn
cucumbers
eggplant
escarole
garlic
ginger root
Jerusalem artichoke
kale
leeks
lettuce (all types)
mushrooms

Vegetables *(cont'd)*

mustard greens
okra
onions
parsley
potatoes
pumpkin
radishes
rutabagas
scallions
shallots
sorrel

spinach
sprouts (all kinds)
squashes (all kinds)
sweet potatoes
Swiss chard
tomatoes
turnips and greens
watercress
yams
zucchini

Fruits

apples
apricots
bananas
blackberries
blueberries
boysenberries
cantaloupe
casaba
cherries
cranberries
currants
dates
figs
grapefruit
grapes
guava
honeydew melon
kiwi fruit
kumquats
lemons

limes
loganberries
mangoes
nectarines
oranges
papayas
peaches
pears
pineapples
plantains
plums
pomegranates
prunes
raisins
raspberries
strawberries
tangelos
tangerines
watermelon

Legumes

All cooked legumes, including:
azuki beans
black beans
black-eyed peas

brown beans
chick-peas (garbanzos)
Great Northern beans
kidney beans

Legumes *(cont'd)*

lentils

miso

mung beans

navy beans

peas

pinto beans

red Mexican beans

soybeans

soy flour

soy milk

split peas

tempeh

tofu

Oils

(1 tablespoon per day)

PREFERRED

safflower oil

ALTERNATIVES

corn oil (unhydrogenated)

walnut oil

sesame oil

sunflower oil

Dairy

nonfat yogurt (plain)

GROUP 2

Fruits

avocado (no more than ¼ per day)

olives (no more than 4 per week)

Nuts and Seeds

(No more than 2 tablespoons of nuts per day, and not more than three times per week.)

almonds

Brazil nuts

cashews

chestnuts

macadamia nuts

peanuts

pecans

pine nuts

pistachio nuts

pumpkin kernels

sesame seeds

sunflower seeds

walnuts

Oils

cottonseed oil

peanut oil

soybean oil

corn oil margarine (tub)

Dairy

nonfat skim milk

GROUP 3

Oils

olive oil   corn oil margarine (stick)

Dairy

low-fat skim milk cheeses   low-fat skim milk
  (uncreamed cottage cheese,   low-fat yogurt
  hoop cheese, farmer cheese,
  mozzarella)

Fish

baked or broiled lean fish

Miscellaneous

egg whites   maple syrup
honey

GROUP 4

Poultry

baked or broiled chicken or
  turkey with skin removed
  before cooking

Fish

all shellfish

Miscellaneous

refined sugar

GROUP 5

Dairy

cream
cream cheeses
whole milk

whole milk cheeses
whole milk yogurt

Meats

all beef products

all pork products

Poultry

fried chicken, with skin

Oil

coconut oil (and coconut)

Miscellaneous

egg yolks

salt

14. How to Eat Well

At first glance, it may seem that a meatless, low-sodium, low-fat diet is one of deprivation. But eating healthfully can be an adventure. And some of your favorite meals are easily adaptable to this way of eating.

During our study, the most popular meal was black-eyed peas and corn bread, coleslaw, and watermelon for dessert. At first, some of the participants grumbled about the absence of salt, and maybe they would have preferred the black-eyed peas with ham hocks. After a while, though, without the salt masking the flavor, they began to taste the beans and the tomatoes, onion, and garlic with which they were cooked.

Of course nobody wants to live on just black-eyed peas and corn bread. But what about spaghetti? or tacos? or stuffed peppers? There are literally hundreds of dishes you can come up with. You do not have to feel like a "health food nut" to eat well.

For example, there are many shapes and sizes of whole grain, eggless pastas to choose from. Whole grain pasta has a much nuttier, richer flavor than white pasta. And meatballs and Alfredo sauce are not the only things with which to toss them. Start with a basic, simple tomato sauce, seasoned with garlic and herbs, and branch out from there. One of the most beautiful and appealing dishes is pasta tossed with steamed vegetables—yellow squash, zucchini, carrots, peas—with parsley or other fresh herbs such as basil and thyme, and sunflower seeds or cracked roasted soybeans (see the recipe on page 221). The colors are vivid, each vegetable tastes distinctive, and the combination of textures—the

149

al dente pasta, the crisp-tender vegetables, and the crunchy sunflower seeds—is superb. If you want to eat very simply, you will never run out of steamed vegetables and salads to try.

Grains and legumes are the staples in this diet. Begin with the familiar ones: rice, kidney beans, lentils, oatmeal. Brown rice has a deeper, more wholesome flavor and a chewier texture than white rice. It takes longer to cook than white rice (unless you use a pressure cooker, a very useful piece of equipment), but it is unsupervised cooking—you don't need to stand over the pot. The same is true for cooking beans. Just put them on the stove and come back when they are ready. Not all beans and grains require a great deal of time; lentils and split peas cook in forty-five minutes, soy flakes in only thirty. Bulgur is cooked just by pouring on boiling water, and couscous (another cracked wheat product) is "cooked" just by pouring on room-temperature water and waiting ten minutes.

Bulgur, couscous, and soy flakes may be new to you—here is where the experience of exploration and discovery begins. You won't have much trouble finding these new foods. More and more supermarkets are stocking them. If you can't find them here, a health food store is likely to have them.

With grains and legumes, you can make salads, soups, casseroles; they can be a side dish or a bed for vegetables or sauces. Grains can even serve as a dessert or as a breakfast cereal. Cooked grains and beans will keep several days in the refrigerator and they freeze well. So, you can always cook more than you need and use the leftovers the next day.

BEGINNING THE TRANSITION

Gradual changes in diet are usually the easiest. Start by reducing your consumption of red meat before you eliminate it altogether. Then, cut down on chicken and fish. Take it one step at a time. As you begin to switch the focus of your diet, begin to experiment with grains and legumes. Cook one vegetarian meal a week, then increase it to two. Introduce yourself to a new grain every so often. If you don't like it the first time, try it again a while later—your tastes might have changed.

Begin by adapting dishes you already enjoy. Rather than go

out and buy new cookbooks, use what is already familiar. Write down a list of your favorite vegetable dishes, including grains, beans, and breads. Include dishes that traditionally contain some meat or cheese, like split pea soup or spinach salad (which usually contain bacon), or lasagne (which usually has cheese and Bolognese sauce), but imagine them without these products.

ADAPTING RECIPES

Begin leafing through your cookbooks. Turn first to vegetables, then look at rice dishes and salads, whole grain baked goods, and grains. Some contain meat, and almost all seem to contain salt, butter, cream, or cheese. That does not rule them out, because they can be modified. If the recipe looks good to you, try it without the salt and the animal products. Use safflower oil instead of butter; you never need more than a tablespoon for sautéing. It is not difficult to sauté vegetables in this amount of oil, especially if you use a nonstick pan; if the pan becomes dry, just add a little water or wine. If something tastes too bland without salt, add herbs, spices, or freshly ground pepper to the dish. At first you may miss the salt, but your palate will quickly adjust.

MODIFYING RECIPES

Remove the meat. If you want to substitute something for texture or bulk, try equivalent measures, in cups, of your choice of cooked grains (such as rice, bulgur, millet, couscous, wheat berries); cooked beans or soy grits; finely chopped steamed vegetables, such as carrots, broccoli, cauliflower, squash, mushrooms (mushrooms are especially meaty); grated carrots; or diced or crumbled tofu.

Remove dairy products. If you wish to replace them, use an equivalent amount of crumbled tofu, or tofu blended with nonfat yogurt.

Use safflower oil, water, or wine in place of butter or any other kinds of oil for cooking. Never use more than 1 tablespoon of safflower oil for sautéing.

Eliminate salt. Experiment with herbs and spices for seasonings.

There are not any good salt substitutes. Salt affects a specific area of your palate, and nothing else will stimulate that area. After a week or so of its absence, though, you will start tasting something else—the food.

We are so used to salt—and it is an acquired addiction—that we have almost forgotten what foods taste like. Vegetables, grains, and legumes all have distinctive, delicious flavors of their own. Salt does not "bring out" their flavors; it interferes with them. But you won't know this until you have stopped using it for a week or two.

Eliminate or substantially reduce the amount of sugar.

Here is an example of how to modify a recipe using these guidelines.

Unmodified Sautéed Eggplant

1–2 large eggplants
salt
3 tablespoons olive oil or butter
1 medium onion, sliced
2 cloves garlic, minced or put through a press
1 green pepper, seeded and diced
¼ cup coarsely chopped almonds
¼ cup coarsely chopped Brazil nuts
¼ cup sunflower seeds
2 tomatoes, peeled and sliced
freshly ground pepper to taste
⅓ cup whole wheat bread crumbs
½ cup grated Parmesan cheese

Slice the eggplants and salt thoroughly. Let sit 30 minutes, then squeeze out moisture and rinse. Squeeze out moisture again and dice.

Heat the oil or butter in a large skillet and sauté the onion, garlic, and green pepper together until the onion begins to soften. Add the eggplant and sauté another 10 minutes. Add the nuts, seeds, and tomatoes and continue to sauté until the eggplant is tender and the mixture aromatic, about 10 to 15 minutes. Season with plenty of salt and ground pepper. Mix together the bread crumbs and the Parmesan and stir into the mixture. Serve.

Modified Sautéed Eggplant

2 eggplants, cut in half lengthwise
2 teaspoons safflower oil, plus additional for baking sheet
1 onion, sliced
2 cloves garlic, minced or put through a press
1 green pepper, seeded and diced
1 cake tofu, diced or crumbled (optional)
3 tablespoons dry white wine
2 tomatoes, peeled and sliced
3 tablespoons sunflower seeds
2 teaspoons chopped fresh basil or 1 teaspoon dried
1 tablespoon chopped fresh parsley
¼ teaspoon allspice or cumin (optional)
½ cup whole wheat bread crumbs
1 tablespoon lime juice, or more to taste
fresh ground pepper

Preheat the oven to 450 degrees. Score the eggplants down to the skin but not through the skin and place on a baking sheet which you have brushed lightly with safflower oil. Bake 20 minutes, until the eggplant is soft. Remove from the heat, and when the eggplant is cool enough to handle, scoop out from the shells and dice.

Heat the 2 teaspoons safflower oil in a heavy-bottomed skillet and sauté the onion, garlic, and green pepper until the onion begins to soften. Add the diced eggplant, the optional tofu, and the white wine and continue to sauté another 5 minutes. Add the tomatoes, sunflower seeds, herbs, bread crumbs, and spices and continue to sauté over medium heat, stirring from time to time, for another 10 to 15 minutes. Add lime juice to taste and grind in plenty of pepper.

For the modified version of this recipe you have eliminated most of the oil, deleted most of the nuts (which are high in fat), and taken out the salt. The wine, herbs, spices, and vegetables will stimulate your palate. The dish is filling, and the tofu adds an additional eight grams of protein.

Most eggplant recipes require salting the eggplant before you sauté it, and when you sauté the eggplant it usually requires a lot of oil and becomes quite saturated. With the method here, the eggplant is "steamed" in a hot oven, which not only draws out the liquid but also brings out its marvelous aroma.

Unmodified Vinaigrette Dressing

    1 tablespoon lemon juice
    3 tablespoons vinegar
    1 clove garlic, minced or put through a press
    1 teaspoon Dijon style mustard
    ¼ teaspoon dried tarragon or 1 teaspoon chopped fresh
        herbs
    ¼ teaspoon salt
    freshly ground pepper to taste
    ¾ cup olive oil

Blend together all the ingredients except the oil. Whisk in the oil.

Modified Vinaigrette Dressing

    juice of ½ lemon
    ¼ cup vinegar
    1 clove garlic, minced or put through a press
    ½ teaspoon dry mustard
    ¼ teaspoon dried tarragon or 1 teaspoon chopped fresh
        herbs
    ¼ teaspoon dried basil or marjoram
    freshly ground pepper to taste
    ½ cup yogurt, water, unsalted tomato juice, or puréed
        tomato
    2 tablespoons safflower oil

Blend together all the ingredients except the safflower oil, and whisk in the oil.

Here you are leaving just enough oil so that the dressing will adhere to the salad. The modified version is just as delicious, with much less fat and no salt. The herbs, vinegar, and lemon juice give it plenty of flavor.

MODIFYING RECIPES CALLING FOR SUGAR

Several foods besides sugar can be used for sweetening dishes. Many desserts are sweet enough without adding anything. Fruits like bananas and baked apples can be puréed in a blender and added to baked goods. Bananas and apple juice can be used to sweeten fruit sherbets, puddings, and tofu pies. Honey, malt syrup, sorghum syrup, and maple syrup also can be used, but only in small quantities.

The Frozen Banana Ice on page 242 is a good example of what can be done. This Dairy Queen-like "ice cream" is made from frozen bananas and a little yogurt. It needs no additional sweetener. Vanilla helps to bring out the sweetness of the bananas, and the dish is further enhanced with nutmeg. Almost all fruits can be transformed into delicious sherberts and frozen ices. Usually you need not add any sweetener, but if, say, the strawberries are not sweet enough, a tablespoon or so of black cherry concentrate (page 164) will go a long way.

Below is a recipe for Bananas Poached in Wine, followed by a modication.

Unmodified Bananas Poached in Wine

    2 cups dry or semi-dry white wine
    ¾ cup sugar
    2 teaspoons vanilla extract
    3-inch stick of cinnamon
    ½ cup raisins or currants
    3–4 firm ripe bananas
    freshly grated nutmeg to taste
    1 cup heavy whipping cream, whipped and flavored with
        vanilla

Combine the white wine, sugar, vanilla, cinnamon, and raisins or currants in a saucepan and bring to a simmer. Stir to dissolve the sugar, cover, and simmer 5 minutes. Peel and slice the bananas and add to the poaching liquid. Cover and simmer 10 minutes. Add nutmeg to taste and serve, topped with whipped cream flavored with vanilla.

Modified Version: Bananas Poached in Apple Juice

2 cups apple juice
1 tablespoon vanilla extract
3-inch stick of cinnamon
¼ cup raisins
3–4 firm ripe bananas
freshly grated nutmeg to taste
½ cup yogurt, flavored with vanilla

Combine the apple juice, vanilla, cinnamon, and raisins in a saucepan and bring to a simmer. Simmer together for 5 minutes. Peel and slice the bananas and add to the poaching liquid. Simmer, covered, for 10 minutes. Add freshly grated nutmeg to taste and serve topped with yogurt flavored with vanilla.

Here the apple juice replaces the wine and sugar combination and produces just as heady a compote. The quantity of raisins has been cut by half, but you will still have raisins to bite into, and the yogurt will give you a nice creamy topping.

If you are used to sweetening your cereals, try adding fresh fruits or a small amount of raisins to them. Another option is to blend up a small amount of yogurt with a banana, or mix together 2 tablespoons of yogurt and 2 tablespoons apple juice and add this to your cereal.

Another easy alternative is to add a few drops of safflower oil to a skillet, heat, and add banana slices, swirling them around until the color becomes amber. They can be served for breakfast instead of bacon—the natural banana oils have a greasy taste, but without the cholesterol. Or, for a tasty dessert, add a little cinnamon, nutmeg, and a dash of rum.

DINING OUT

Every kind of restaurant has healthful food for you. Oriental restaurants almost always have a variety of vegetarian meals. Italian restaurants have pastas with tomato sauce or vegetables, salads, vegetable side dishes, and fruit desserts. Continental restaurants often serve rice and vegetable side dishes, as well as a variety of salads. And there are always rice, beans, tortillas, and salads at Mexican restaurants. Even a steak house will serve a baked potato and vegetables, and many have a salad bar.

When you go to a restaurant, look through the entire menu first. Vegetable dishes are usually scattered throughout. An easy strategy is to order two dishes from the hors d'oeuvre section, and ask the waiter to bring one selection as a first course and the second selection as an entrée. If you don't see anything you think you can eat on the menu, ask the waiter if the chef can do something special for you. Almost any restaurant will make a fruit plate or vegetable plate for you, even if it is not on the menu. Restaurants always have vegetables on hand, and it usually will not inconvenience them to cook some for you. Or, for instance, if you are in an Italian restaurant and you don't see any vegetarian entrées, ask the chef to cook some plain pasta for you and toss it with some vegetables. Order a big salad to go with this, with the dressing on the side, and you have a complete meal.

If you know where you are going to be dining, call ahead. Find out if they have anything suitable on their menu, or if they could do something special for you. Ask them to leave out the salt, excess oil, eggs, and animal products. Many chefs, especially in high-quality restaurants, will consider this an interesting challenge.

If you can't find an entrée on the menu, the chef won't cooperate, and everything looks hopeless, simply order a big salad with the dressing on the side, some vegetables, and an unbuttered potato. Ask the cook not to sauté the vegetables in butter. If you are ordering a large salad, ask the waiter to bring it without the items that you don't want (such as eggs, anchovies, or bacon).

Another concern is that your friends will feel uncomfortable about inviting you to dinner or that they have to go out of their way for you. No one will feel uncomfortable if you avoid proselytizing. At a large dinner party, simply eat whatever side dishes are available. When invited to a smaller dinner, it is usually best to mention your dietary preferences to the host or hostess beforehand, so they will not be offended when you don't eat some of the dishes they might be serving. Reassure them that they need not cook a special meal—the side dishes and vegetables they are serving will be plenty. And again, to be sure, you might have a bite to eat before you leave your house.

EQUIPMENT

This diet requires no new fancy equipment. If you have a couple of good knives, a few pots and pans, a soup pot, and a baking dish, you already have what you need. The items below can make time spent in the kitchen a little more efficient and enjoyable, but most of them are not essential.

Pots and Pans

If you want to invest in some helpful items, begin with some good nonstick cookware. Some of the heavier Silverstone pots and pans are especially useful. With these, you can sauté with virtually no oil, yet grains do not stick to the saucepans. Whatever cookware you use, begin with two or three saucepans (two- or four-quart), a soup pot or Dutch oven, and a 10-inch or 12-inch skillet.

Pressure Cooker. This reduces cooking times for beans by more than one-half. Use it for all beans except soybeans, split peas, lentils, and soy flakes; these bubble up too much and will clog the pressure cooker.

Slow Cooker. These also facilitate bean cookery, as well as that of grains and soups. Just put all the ingredients into the slow cooker, turn it on low or medium, and forget about it for hours. You can put in your beans and water in the morning, go to work, and when you come home dinner will be waiting.

Steamer. Stainless steel fold-up steamers are inexpensive and indispensable for steaming vegetables.

Wok. To sauté vegetables.

A Large Pot for Pasta. This can be an inexpensive enameled pan, such as the kind used for canning. (I use an old baby bottle sterilizer I bought at a secondhand store.)

Utensils

Knives. A food processor is not necessary for most kitchen tasks. What is necessary is a good set of kitchen knives, and a sharpening stone and steel for keeping them sharp. Dull knives make chopping vegetables a time-consuming chore—and a dangerous one—since they tend to slip off whatever you are cutting and onto your finger.

You will need an 8-inch stainless steel or carbon steel knife and a paring knife. Carbon steel remains sharp longer than stainless steel. A stainless steel knife is best for cutting fruit, as carbon steel will become discolored because of the acid, giving the fruit a metallic taste. A serrated bread knife is also helpful.

At least two wooden spoons
Whisk
Metal spatula
Plastic or rubber spatula
Four-sided grater
Nutmeg grater, for fresh nutmeg
Garlic press
Pepper mill
Citrus juicer
Bread board for kneading and rolling out dough
Rolling pin
Colander
Strainer
Lettuce dryer
Kitchen timer
Potato peeler
At least three mixing bowls

Measures

2-cup Pyrex measuring cup
4-cup Pyrex measuring cup
Set of individual measuring cups
One or two sets of measuring spoons

Baking Dishes

A three- or four-quart baking dish or casserole
A one- or two-quart baking dish or casserole
One or two 9- or 10-inch pie pans

Two nonstick bread pans
Two nonstick 12-muffin tins
Two or three nonstick baking sheets with rims
Two 10-inch pizza pans (baking sheets can be used instead)

Electrical Appliances

Blender
Electric Mixer. Not essential, but if you have one with a dough hook, it can save time with breadmaking.

Food Processor. As long as you have a blender, you do not need a food processor. They are handy for making pâtés and some sauces, and for puréeing vegetables, although all of this can be done with a blender in a little more time. Only two recipes in this collection require a food processor: the Frozen Banana Ice (see page 242) and Mixed Fruit Ice (see page 279).

Sorbettier or Electric Ice Cream Maker. Although these appliances can be expensive and are not essential, either an electric ice cream freezer or a sorbettier (an electric aerator that fits into your freezer) will allow you to make all kinds of fruit ices with very little work.

GLOSSARY OF INGREDIENTS

Most of the components of this diet are available in your supermarket. The exception will be some of the grains, whole grain flours, beans, and a few specialty items such as fruit concentrates and nut butters; these are available in most health food stores. It is economical and convenient to buy grains in these stores, especially if you are just beginning to cook with these foods, because you can buy only the amount called for in a recipe. On the other hand, items such as apple juice are usually much less expensive in a supermarket, and no less healthful.

The list below is by no means exhaustive. It includes the items in the recipes that follow. Grains, legumes, and flours should be stored in labeled, airtight jars. Keep grains and beans in a cool, dry place. It is best to refrigerate flours, since their oils are quite volatile. Refrigerate all oils, nuts, and seeds.

Grains (See also Chapter 15 for general cooking instructions.)

Brown Rice. Both short grain and long grain are available. Very versatile. Both take about 40 to 45 minutes to cook.

Wild Rice. This is actually a grass. The grains are long, light, and delicate, with a particularly savory flavor. It makes excellent pilafs, but is very expensive because of its rarity and the difficulty with which it is harvested.

Millet. Small, round, yellow grain that has a delicate, nutty flavor when cooked. Takes about 40 minutes to cook. Can be substituted for brown rice in most recipes, and also makes a nice breakfast cereal.

Bulgur. A cracked wheat cereal that has been precooked, then dehydrated. A very convenient food—to prepare it, simply pour on boiling water and let it sit for 20 to 30 minutes. You can also let it soak overnight or for several hours in a marinade, for luscious cracked wheat salads (see Tabbouleh, page 250). Bulgur is tawny brown in color and has a rich, nutty taste.

Couscous. Another cracked wheat cereal product which has been partially cooked and dehydrated. Couscous is made from hard semolina wheat and is light yellow, almost white in color. You can cook it in 10 minutes, just by adding some warm water to rehydrate it. It has the most delicate, silky texture of all the grains, and a subtle flavor.

Cracked Wheat. A cracked wheat cereal that has not been precooked. Takes about 30 minutes to cook in simmering water, and has a slightly harder texture than bulgur, but a similar nutty taste. Particularly good in breads.

Barley. Looks somewhat like brown rice, though a little lighter in color. It becomes puffier when it cooks and has a pleasing, chewing consistency and a satisfying flavor. Especially good in soups and pilafs. It was made to go with mushrooms, as in Mushroom and Barley Soup (see page 270).

Whole Wheat Berries. These look like a dark brown version of brown rice. Wheat flour is milled from wheat berries. They take about 50 to 60 minutes to cook and have a very chewy, almost meaty consistency.

Whole Rye. These look like wheat berries but are a little longer and thinner. They take about 50 to 60 minutes to cook and have a rich, almost salty flavor. They go nicely with cara-way seeds, as all lovers of rye bread know.

Flaked or Rolled Oats. High in protein, a marvelous breakfast cereal, and also great in breads. Cook in only about 10 to 15 minutes.

Flaked Wheat. These look like a darker version of flaked oats and have a chewier flavor. Have them for breakfast as a variation on oatmeal.

Flaked Rye. Like flaked oats, but darker and chewier, with a distinctive rye flavor.

Triticale. This is a hybrid of wheat and rye, developed in the last twenty years. It is high in protein and has a rich flavor of its own. The whole berries can be used interchangeably with wheat and rye, while the flakes can be used interchangeably with oats, wheat, and rye. When milled, it is a distinctive flavor for bread.

Flours

Whole wheat
Whole wheat pastry
Unbleached white
Rye
Soy
Stone-ground corn meal
Wheat germ
Triticale flour
Masa Harina. A special kind of corn flour, for which corn kernels have been soaked in a lime solution. It is the basis for corn tortillas.

Legumes (See also Chapter 15 for general cooking instructions.)

Azuki Beans. Small red Japanese beans. A somewhat sweet taste.

Black Beans. A favorite. These have a rich, savory flavor and are terrific as a topping for chalupas or nachos or as a filling for enchiladas.

Black-eyed Peas. Another popular bean. These seem to be better known in the South, where it is the custom to eat them for good luck on New Year's Day. A comforting flavor.

Garbanzos or Chick-peas. One and the same. These beans have a truly distinctive flavor. You may think you don't like this tasty legume if you are only accustomed to the salad bar variety, since salad bars often utilize canned garbanzos that lose their texture and become mealy.

Kidney Beans. The familiar kidney-shaped red bean that is often used in salads and soups.

Lentils. Another well-known food, they are delicious in soups and marinated salads. They cook quickly (about 45 minutes) and require no soaking. You can cook them in the same pot with rice for a balanced, filling dish. They make delicious sprouts.

Lima Beans. Dried lima beans are less mealy than fresh ones.

Mung Beans. Used primarily for sprouts: high in protein and low in calories and fat.

Navy Beans, Small White Beans, Cannellini. These are three different varieties of white beans, all of which can be used interchangeably. They have a subtle flavor and make marvelous soups, salads, and spreads.

Peanuts. Familiar to everyone.

Pinto Beans. Larger than black beans, speckled light brown in color.

Soybeans. A very important food because of their high protein content.

Soy Flakes. Soybeans that have been cooked, split, and dehydrated. Very convenient—they cook in about 30 minutes and can be cooked along with grains for balanced protein.

Soy Grits. These are cracked soybeans and look somewhat like cracked wheat. They are also very convenient because they cook more quickly than soybeans and can be cooked along with grains. They have a rather crunchy texture and nutty taste.

Seeds

Because nuts are so high in fat, they don't have much of a place in this diet. However, there are a few seeds which, although high in fat, can be included for texture and flavor.

Alfalfa Seeds. Used to make sprouts, which can substitute for lettuce in sandwiches (and they don't wilt like lettuce does), they make a nice garnish for salads and soups, and they make good salads on their own.

Chia Seeds. These tiny black seeds are very high in protein. When soaked in water, they become viscous and take on some of the properties of egg whites, adding lightness and protein to baked goods.

Flax Seeds. These resemble sesame seeds in appearance, except they are dark brown and shiny (very pretty). Like chia, but even more so, they have a magical property when soaked in water: they become viscous like egg whites and are a useful ingredient in baked goods that traditionally contain eggs.

Sesame Seeds. Add flavor and texture to many dishes.

Sunflower Seeds. Add flavor and crunch to a variety of dishes.

Oil

The only oil used in these recipes is safflower oil. It is the highest in polyunsaturates and has a mild, all-purpose unobtrusive flavor.

Pasta

Whole grain pastas come in several varieties of flour combinations, such as whole wheat/sesame, whole wheat/soy, sesame/soy, spinach/sesame, regular whole wheat, buckwheat (also known as soba), and more. There are many sizes to choose from, and almost all are made without eggs or salt. Consult the package to be sure. Pastas look beautiful when stored in tightly covered, tall jars.

Sweeteners

Apple Concentrate. A very concentrated apple juice that can be used to sweeten some dishes.

Black Cherry Concentrate. A sweet concentrate made from black cherries; used to sweeten some desserts. A little goes a long way.

Mild-Flavored Honeys. Choose light-colored varieties for the mildest flavor—clover honeys, acacia, lavender, and wildflower.

Malt Syrup. This is a thick syrup made from sprouted barley. It has a delightful, mild flavor, not as sweet as honey, and it is higher in trace vitamins and minerals.

Sorghum Syrup. Another thick syrup, this tastes like a very mild-flavored molasses and is rich in minerals.

Maple Syrup. Look for pure maple syrup.

Herbs and Spices

Herbs and spices are almost essential to a low-sodium diet. They divert your palate in its search for salt by accenting food with their unique flavors. Small quantities can transform the nature of a dish and bring it alive in a completely new way. Fresh basil, for example, makes tomato sauces and soups (like the Gazpacho on page 249) many times more interesting. Fresh coriander (also known as cilantro) enhances beans and Mexican and Oriental dishes with its distinctive flavor. Caraway is another singular tasting herb. It is particularly pleasing in rye breads and in the Potato-Caraway Salad on page 244. Cumin is often used in Mexican and Indian foods and as a seasoning for more simple vegetable preparations.

One of the simplest and most satisfying ways to use herbs, fresh or dried, is to accent steamed vegetables. One to two tablespoons of chopped fresh herbs (or a teaspoon of dried) can transform four servings of vegetables.

Most herbs are easy to grow if you have a little sun. An apartment window or terrace is enough space for a few small pots. If you don't grow your own herbs and can't find fresh ones, dried herbs are fine.

You may find the flavors of some herbs and spices unfamiliar at first. Because their characteristics are unique, they may surprise your palate. Try them more than once, for you may grow fond of some even though you may not like them immediately. If you prefer your food very simple, just omit the herbs and spices.

Below is a list of the herbs and spices that will occur in the recipes in this collection. It is by no means exhaustive.

HERBS

Anise. Has a licorice-like flavor. It is usually the seeds that are used. Particularly good in sweet breads and can also make a nice addition to gazpacho.

Basil. Sweet and vaguely like anise, though less of a licorice taste. It is marvelous in many Italian dishes and was made to accompany tomatoes.

Bay Leaves. Subtle and savory, they enhance soups and beans, especially lentils and white beans.

Caraway. The seeds have a distinctive flavor that can give breads (especially rye) and other dishes a new dimension.

Cayenne. Very hot. A little goes a long way, and a pinch can accent a dish without overpowering it.

Chili Powder. There are many kinds, varying in degree of piquancy from mild to hot. Be careful to check labels, because salt is often added. You can make your own by grinding up dried chili peppers in a spice mill.

Cilantro or Fresh Coriander. Also called Chinese parsley, since it looks sort of like flat Italian parsley and is often found in Oriental dishes. Its flavor is spicy and strong. Great with beans and in other Mexican dishes.

Coriander. The dried seeds, cracked or ground, have a very different taste from their fresh counterpart. It is a spicy taste, though not hot, and it enhances vegetables in an interesting way. It is one of the ingredients in curry powder.

Cumin. Ground cumin seeds are a must in Mexican dishes and curries, but they also make a marvelous seasoning for steamed vegetables, vegetable pâtés, salad dressings, and salads like the Tabbouleh on page 250.

Dill. Fresh dill is perfect for dishes like Marinated Cucumber Salad (page 279), and is a delicious seasoning for steamed vegetables like carrots, squash, and potatoes. It never overpowers a dish, yet it has a special flavor. Dill salad dressings are terrific.

Dill Seed. In the seed form dill is similar to, but not as strong as, caraway. It is tasty in breads and salad dressings.

Garlic. Use fresh garlic whenever possible; the powdered form is often stale and unappetizing. Garlic is very pungent in its raw state but becomes quite mild as it cooks.

Marjoram. Delicious on salads. It is related to oregano and has a minty, oregano-like flavor. The dried form enhances most salad dressings and steamed vegetables.

Mints. Fresh mints, such as peppermint, spearmint, or pennyroyal, can transform an ordinary fruit dessert into a sensational one. There are a number of varieties, and most are easy to grow. Blend a few sprigs of mint with a glass of orange juice or apple juice to make a particularly refreshing drink.

Parsley. Probably the fresh herb with which most people are familiar. It goes with a variety of vegetables, grains, and beans.

Rosemary. This herb has a savory, woody flavor. It is very distinctive and goes well with vegetables like tomatoes, mushrooms, and summer squash.

Sage. Goes well with potatoes, if used sparingly.

Tarragon. Sweet and delicate, especially good in salad dressings and some sauces. It is difficult to find fresh, but the dried form is good.

Thyme. Another savory herb that goes well with mushrooms, tomatoes, and many other vegetables, as well as with grains and dried beans.

SPICES

Allspice. A sweet spice that accompanies cinnamon in many dishes.

Cardamom. Has a unique flavor that enhances fruits in an interesting way. It also is used in curries.

Cinnamon. Familiar to all. A pinch or two will bring out the savory flavors of an Italian tomato sauce.

Cloves. A sweet and pungent spice that is a major ingredient in chutneys and relishes.

Curry Powder. This is actually a mixture of spices and chilies, and the "hotness" can vary. The major seasoning for Indian dishes.

Ginger. Fresh ginger is delicious in Oriental dishes, some sauces, and some desserts. It is pungent and somewhat sharp. Dried ginger has a more concentrated character than fresh.

Mace. A sweet spice which falls in the cinnamon, all-spice, and nutmeg category.

Nutmeg. Freshly grated nutmeg is more distinctive than the ground nutmeg you buy at the store.

Black Peppercorns. Freshly ground pepper will probably find its way into your diet much more often after you eliminate salt.

Red Pepper Flakes or Dried Red Peppers. There are many different kinds of peppers, each with its own unique flavor. They are all hot, some more so than others. The flakes are the hottest part.

Turmeric. A component in curry powders that gives foods a pretty yellow hue. It has a mildly bitter flavor.

Miscellaneous

Arrowroot Powder. A thickening agent like cornstarch. It is used in some of the sauces in this collection.

Postum. A rich grain beverage that can be used as a coffee substitute. Dark and somewhat sweet.

Sesame Tahini. Raw sesame butter, made from ground sesame seeds.

Instant Soy Milk (such as Fearn or Jolly Joan). Although not particularly appealing by itself, it can be used in recipes that normally call for milk, such as the Millet Raisin Pudding on page 277. Flavored with a little vanilla and apple juice, it isn't bad with cereal. Soy milk can be found in health food stores.

Spray-Dried Milk. A concentrated form of dried milk, twice as concentrated as instant varieties like Carnation. Used for making nonfat yogurt. There is virtually no fat in nonfat, spray-dried milk such as Sanalac. Found in most supermarkets.

Tofu. Also known as bean curd, a type of soy cheese made from soy milk. Found in most supermarkets. It is very bland by itself, but because of its soft, porous texture it absorbs flavors readily. If you dice it up and cook it in a curry dish, it will be curry-flavored; if you cook it with tomatoes it will have a rich, tomato flavor. Tofu is very versatile; it can be crumbled into salads, diced and cooked in mixed vegetable dishes, and blended into sauces. It can also be puréed and baked into cheesecakes and pies, like the Tofu Banana Cream Pie on page 246. Tofu is high in protein, moderate in fat, inexpensive, and versatile.

Unsweetened Preserves and Fruit Spreads. Some of the most common are unsweetened apple butter and apricot butter. Found in most whole foods stores. You can also make some yourself (see recipes for Plum Sauce [page 208] and Apricot Preserves [page 193]. Arrowhead Mills has a whole line of unsweetened fruit spreads—boysenberry, blackberry, strawberry, raspberry, apple, combinations like apple-strawberry.

15. General Cooking Instructions for Grains, Legumes, and Vegetables

The recipes that follow are the ones to master first. They are the foundation for this cuisine. Once you understand the basics, the range of possibilities for this diet become endless. If you know how to cook grains and beans, how to steam vegetables, and how to make some simple sauces, then dinner will never be a problem. With these items, some bread, and a salad, lunch or a light supper will always be on hand.

GENERAL COOKING DIRECTIONS FOR GRAINS

One cup of grain feeds four people.

Brown Rice, Barley, Soy Grits

Use 1 part grain to 2 parts water. Combine the grain and water in a saucepan and bring to a boil. Reduce heat, cover, and simmer 35 minutes until most of the liquid is absorbed. Remove the lid and cook, uncovered, for 5 to 10 minutes longer, to separate the grains. (Soy grits are not a grain, but they cook in the same way as brown rice.)

Millet

Use 1 part millet to 2½ parts water. Heat 1 teaspoon safflower oil in a saucepan and sauté the millet until it begins to smell toasty and the grains are coated with oil (about 3 to 5 minutes).

Add the water and bring to a boil. Reduce heat, cover, and simmer 35 minutes. Remove the lid and continue to simmer until the liquid is evaporated (about 10 more minutes).

Buckwheat Groats (Kasha)

Use 1 part groats, 2 parts water. Use the same method as for cooking millet (above).

Wheat Berries, Whole Rye, Triticale

Use 1 part grain, 3 parts water. Combine the grain and water and bring to a boil. Reduce heat, cover, and simmer for 50 minutes. Remove from the heat and pour off any excess liquid.

Bulgur

Use 1 part bulgur to 2 parts water. Place the bulgur in a bowl. Bring the water to a boil and pour over the bulgur. Let it sit until the water is absorbed and the bulgur is soft and fluffy (about 20 to 30 minutes). Pour off the excess water and squeeze bulgur dry in a cheesecloth or dish towel. (Bulgur also can be soaked for a longer time in a dressing, as in the Tabbouleh recipe on page 250.)

Couscous

Use 1 part couscous to 2 parts lukewarm water. Pour the water over the couscous and allow it to sit for 10 minutes. Fluff with a fork.

Additions for Flavoring Grains

All of these grains can be prepared with seasonings and vegetables to give them more flavor. Simply combine the additions with the water and grains and cook according to the directions.

several cloves garlic, cut in thick slices
1 onion, chopped
1 carrot, chopped

fresh or dried herbs, such as thyme, rosemary, oregano, basil, marjoram, dill, caraway (caraway is especially good with whole rye and triticale). Use ½ teaspoon per cup of grain (more to taste).

spices such as cumin, curry powder, ginger, paprika, chili powder

2 tablespoons raisins or currants per cup grains

juice of ½ lemon per cup grains

GENERAL COOKING DIRECTIONS FOR LEGUMES

Several of the dishes in this book call for cooked beans. This requires a bit of foresight, as the beans must be soaked first and take up to two hours to cook, unless you have a pressure cooker. Refer to the cooking directions below, using whichever soaking method you prefer, for preparing beans called for in the recipes that follow.

If you want to have cooked beans on hand, cook twice as much as you need each time you make a batch, and freeze half in 1-cup batches (zip-lock bags make good containers). They will take about 1 hour to thaw.

If your beans seem to take hours and hours to cook, it may be that your water is hard. In this case, try using bottled water.

Note that one cup of beans feeds three people.

Soaking Method 1. Wash and pick over the beans, making sure there are no little stones masquerading as beans. Soak the beans in 3 times their volume of water for at least 6 hours in the refrigerator.

Soaking Method 2. With this method you'll never have to worry about forgetting to soak the beans. Wash and pick over the beans. Place in a pot with 3 times their volume of water and bring to a rolling boil. Boil 2 minutes, then cover tightly and turn off the heat. Let sit for 2 hours and proceed with the recipe.

Very Simple Cooked Beans

Some beans, such as garbanzos and soybeans, have such a distinctive flavor of their own that they can be cooked with no further seasonings. Also, if you are using the beans in another dish that will be adequately seasoned, you need not go to the trouble of making Savory Beans (see next recipe). Use 1 part beans, washed, picked over, and soaked (use Method 1 or 2), to 3 parts water.

Combine the beans and water in a saucepan or bean pot that is at least their volume and bring to a boil. (The size of the pot is especially important with soybeans, which bubble up dramatically.) Cover, reduce heat, and simmer 1 to 2 hours until tender.

Savory Beans

Garlic and onions are the key to a good pot of beans. Other herbs and vegetables also will increase the flavor. Peppers, either sweet or hot, will pep up a pot of black beans or pinto beans and give it a Mexican flair; fresh coriander (cilantro) is another welcome addition to these two varieties of beans, as are cumin and chili powder. White beans and lentils are always enhanced by bay leaves and parsley, and tomatoes are an excellent accompaniment to black-eyed peas.

Basic Savory Beans, Method 1

2 teaspoons safflower oil
1 large onion, chopped
3–4 cloves garlic, minced or put through a press
2 cups beans, washed, picked over, and soaked
6 cups water

Heat the oil in a heavy-bottomed soup pot or Dutch oven and sauté the onion and half the garlic until the onion is tender. Add the beans and water and bring to a boil. Add any additional ingredients (see Additions sections on the next page). Cover, reduce heat, and simmer 30 minutes. Add the remaining garlic and continue to simmer, covered, for another hour, or until tender.

Note: Lentils and split peas take only about 45 minutes.

Basic Savory Beans, Method 2

Omit the safflower oil. Place all the ingredients in a pot, bring to a boil, and proceed as in Method 1, simmering, covered, until tender.

Pressure-Cooked Beans

Use Method 1 or 2, up to the point where the beans come to a boil. Then cover and bring to 15 pounds pressure. Reduce the heat to medium and cook 30 minutes for soaked beans, 60 for unsoaked.

Remove from the heat and run the pressure cooker under cold water for several minutes. Remove the gauge, and when all the steam has been released, carefully remove the lid. Do not remove the lid until all the steam has escaped.

Slow-Cooked Beans

These can be cooked either in a slow cooker or in the oven. To cook in the oven, place all the ingredients plus 2 additional cups water in an ovenproof bean pot or casserole, cover, and set in a 200- to 220-degree oven (low setting). Close the oven door and leave all day or all night. You will have a thick, soupy, tender pot of beans after 6 to 8 hours.

Additions for Flavoring Beans

To enhance the flavor of black beans and pintos (2 cups, uncooked), use any one or a combination of the following ingredients:

    2–3 tablespoons fresh coriander (cilantro)
    1–3 teaspoons ground cumin
    1–3 teaspoons chili powder
    1 bell pepper, chopped
    2 jalapeños, cut in half, seeds removed
    1 bay leaf
    1–2 oranges, cut in half or left whole
    3–4 tablespoons dry sherry

Additions for Flavoring Lentils, Split Peas, White Beans, Black-eyed Peas, and Garbanzos

To enhance the flavor of lentils, split peas, and other legumes, use one or more of the following ingredients:

additional garlic
1 bay leaf
2 sprigs parsley
1 sprig fresh rosemary or ¼–½ teaspoon dried
2 sprigs fresh tyme or ¼–½ teaspoon dried
3 leaves fresh sage or a pinch of dried
2–3 chopped fresh tomatoes
½–1 teaspoon dried oregano
½–1 teaspoon dried basil
1 carrot, chopped
1 dried hot red pepper or a pinch of cayenne
1–2 teaspoons paprika

Cooked Soy Flakes

Use 1 part soy flakes and 2½ parts water. Bring the water to a boil in a pot which is at least twice the volume of the flakes and water, and add the soy flakes. Bring to a second boil, reduce heat, and simmer 30 minutes. Drain excess liquid. Season with lime juice.

GENERAL COOKING DIRECTIONS FOR VEGETABLES

Steaming vegetables allows them to retain their color, texture, and many of their water-soluble vitamins.

Place the vegetables in a stainless steel or bamboo steamer (on top of a plate if your steamer allows) above 1 or 2 inches of water in a saucepan. Putting the vegetables on a plate or bowl allows you to save the liquid that escapes as they cook. You can then use this liquid in a sauce, soup, or dressing (or even drink it). Bring the water to a boil, cover the pot, and reduce the heat.

Vegetables vary in their steaming times. Steam green vegetables, squash, cauliflower, and turnips for 5 to 10 minutes, then refresh them under cold water to stop the cooking, or serve them right away, piping hot.

Artichokes and root vegetables take longer. Artichokes take 45 minutes to 1 hour. Carrots cut in sticks and small turnips quartered take about 10 to 15 minutes, and beets and potatoes can take anywhere from 20 to 40 minutes, depending on their size. To hasten the cooking time you can cut them into smaller pieces.

If you are just starting out with steaming, experiment. You can always put something back and cook it some more.

Cooking Eggplant

Most eggplant recipes require salting the eggplant before you sauté it, and when you do sauté the eggplant, it always seems to require a lot of oil and becomes quite saturated. With the method given here, the eggplant is "steamed" in a hot oven, which not only draws out the liquid but also brings out its marvelous aroma.

Preheat the oven to 450 degrees. Cut the eggplant in half lengthwise. With a sharp knife make two lengthwise slits in each half, cutting through *to* the skin but not through it. Brush a baking sheet with safflower oil and place the eggplant on it cut side down. Pop it into the oven for 20 minutes or until the skins begin to shrivel. Remove from the oven and allow to cool. The eggplant will be soft and fragrant. When cool enough to handle, proceed with your recipe.

16. Bread

Every meal can be filling and easy with the addition of a whole grain bread. The only trouble is that it is often difficult to find unsalted bread. Recently there have been more brands of whole grain, low-sodium bread appearing on the market, but it's always good to have a recipe of your own.

The recipes that follow are easy. Making bread may seem like a mystery if you have never done it, but it really isn't too formidable a task. Most of the mystery revolves around its rising, but given sufficient kneading and a warm location, almost any yeasted dough will rise.

GENERAL DIRECTIONS FOR
BREAD BAKING

Mixing the Dough. First dissolve the yeast in some of the water, according to the recipe. It will begin to foam or proof in about 10 minutes, and you can proceed with the recipe. If it does not, the yeast is no longer active and you must begin again with new yeast. You usually mix together the wet ingredients, then fold or beat in the dry, until you can turn the mixture out of the bowl in a semblance of a mass, and knead.

Sometimes the first step is a "sponge." This is a mixture of the yeast, sweetener, water, and half the flour, which rises for an hour before you mix in the remaining ingredients and knead. It gets the yeast moving before the heavy grains and flours arrive to slow it down.

176

Kneading. Once the dough can be turned out of the bowl in more or less one piece, place a half cup of flour on your kneading surface and turn out the dough. Don't worry if some of the dough adheres to the bowl; just scrape what adheres out onto the dough.

Flour your hands and remove your rings before starting to knead. Gently fold the mass of dough in half toward you. Using the "heels" of your hands, lean into it. The pressure should flatten out the dough. Then turn the dough a quarter turn. Fold it in half and lean into it again. Continue the fold, lean, turn rhythm for about 10 minutes. At first the dough will be sticky, and you will have to add handfuls of flour to your board whenever it begins to stick. The dough will begin to stiffen up after the first few turns.

After 10 minutes of kneading, the dough should be elastic as well as stiff. When adding flour, add as little as possible. Always make any necessary additions to the board, not to the dough. Shape into a ball by turning and folding four times without leaning into it. Pinch the underside together to make a seam.

Oil the bowl, and place the dough in it seam side up first, to coat the surface with oil, then seam side down. Cover with plastic or a towel and set in a warm place to rise until double in bulk.

Rising. This usually takes 1 to 1½ hours. A warm place can be over a pilot light (if the light isn't too hot), in an oven with a pilot light, in an oven which has been turned on low for 10 minutes and then turned off, or even in the sun. In summer an un-air-conditioned kitchen is usually warm enough.

Punching Down. Simply stick your fist into the center of the dough several times. Some breadmakers like to test the dough before punching down to see if it has risen enough. This can be done by gently pressing a finger into the dough. If the well caused by the depression does not fill in, then sufficient time has passed for rising.

Shaping Loaves. Most of the breads in this collection do not rise in the bowl again after punching down. To shape a loaf, press the dough out into a rectangle, about as wide as the bread pan is long, and either fold up like a business letter or roll up like a log. Pinch the lengthwise seam together, fold the ends over toward the crease, and pinch the folds.

Oil your bread pans and place the loaves in them, seam side up first. Press into the pans to shape, then turn the loaves over so that the seam side is down. Cover with a towel and let rise in a warm place until they have risen above the edges of the pan. Meanwhile preheat the oven.

Some breads have to be scored with a knife to prevent them from splitting during baking. Others do not. See recipes for instructions.

Bake until the crust is golden brown and the bread responds to tapping with a hollow thumping sound. Remove from the pans and cool on racks.

Storing. Bread should be double-wrapped: in plastic and foil, in plastic and a plastic bag, or in two plastic bags. It can then be refrigerated or frozen.

Using an Electric Mixer

All of the recipes which follow can be made in an electric mixer with a dough hook. The procedure is a little different.

1. Dissolve the yeast in some of the water according to the recipe, to proof.

2. Combine the dry ingredients except the last 2 cups flour in the mixing bowl. Mix together with the dough hook on the second speed.

3. Combine the liquid ingredients and gradually add to the flour mixture, along with the yeast, beating on speed 2.

4. Continue beating on speed 2, adding the remaining flour, ½ cup at a time, as necessary. Continue to mix about 5 minutes.

5. When dough clings to hook, or hook sweeps around center of the dough leaving a clean cylinder and the dough knocks against the sides of the bowl, knead on speed 2 for 7 to 10 minutes, until dough is elastic and fairly smooth (it will still be a little sticky).

6. Remove dough hook, cover dough, and proceed with the recipe.

Note: Many instruction books for mixers say that dough should cling to the hook and clean the sides of the bowl. Whole grain breads don't always do this, but it shouldn't worry you. As long as the hook comes in contact with the dough, it is being kneaded.

Using a Food Processor

Many breads can be made in a food processor. Depending on the size of your machine, you can make up to 2 loaves, though a 1-loaf recipe is usually easier to deal with. Use the short plastic blade that comes with the machine. Proof the yeast in ½ cup water with a small amount of honey. When it is bubbly, pour into your food processor bowl. Add the remaining water and other liquid ingredients. Add the rest of the ingredients. Knead by using the pulse action of the machine, stopping and starting for about 5 minutes. Do not overknead; stop when the blades begin to tear the dough and it does not remain in a lump. Remove the dough from the food processor bowl, transfer to an oiled bowl, cover, and let rise in a warm spot. Proceed with the directions in the recipe.

Herbed Triticale Bread
Makes 1 loaf

This is a superb bread. Because of the savory flavor of the herbs and onion and the nutty, rich taste of the triticale, you won't miss the salt. And it's easy to make. The dough, which is sticky, requires an hour-long rise, then a 40-minute rise in the pan. It bakes in 50 minutes. It slices well, and it can be frozen.

    1 tablespoon active dry yeast
    ½ cup lukewarm water
    1 tablespoon mild-flavored honey
    2 tablespoons plus 1 teaspoon safflower oil, plus additional
    ½ medium onion, minced
    1 cup Homemade Nonfat Yogurt (page 217)
    1½ cups triticale flour (substitute rye if you can't find
        triticale)
    1 tablespoon dried dill
    1 tablespoon dill seed
    1 teaspoon dried sage
    3 cups whole wheat flour

In a large bowl, dissolve the yeast in the warm water and add the honey. Let it stand 10 minutes. Meanwhile, heat 1 teaspoon of the safflower oil in a skillet and sauté the onion until tender. Remove from the heat and cool.

When the yeat is bubbly, stir in the remaining 2 tablespoons safflower oil, the yogurt, triticale flour, dill, dill seed, and sage. Beat well and begin to fold in the whole wheat flour.

Because the dough is sticky, it can be kneaded right in the bowl. Add the whole wheat flour a cup at a time and fold in. When you have added all 3 cups, knead the dough in the bowl for about 10 minutes. Or you can put the third cup of flour on your board and turn out the dough. It will be sticky, but just keep flouring your hands and knead quickly. Use a pastry scraper if you wish to scrape the dough off the board and fold it over.

Oil your bowl; place the dough in it seam side up first, then seam side down. Cover the bowl tightly and let rise in a warm place for 1 hour, until almost doubled in bulk. Flour your fist (as the dough will be sticky) and punch down.

Oil a bread pan or a 2-quart soufflé dish. If using a soufflé dish or pan that isn't well seasoned, you should line it with parchment. Form the dough into a loaf (or a ball for the soufflé dish) and place it in the pan. Make three ½-inch-deep slashes across the surface and let the dough rise for 40 minutes in a warm place. Preheat the oven to 350 degrees 10 minutes before the end of the rising time. Bake in the preheated oven for 50 minutes, or until the loaves are brown and respond to tapping with a hollow thumping sound. Remove from the pan and cool on a rack.

Whole Wheat Sage and Onion Bread
Makes 1 loaf

This is a tasty bread because of the onion and sage. And it's as easy to make as the preceding triticale bread.

    2 tablespoons active dry yeast
    ½ cup lukewarm water
    2 tablespoons plus ½ teaspoon mild-flavored honey
    1 cup Homemade Nonfat Yogurt (page 217)
    2 tablespoons grated onion
    2 teaspoons dried sage
    2 tablespoons safflower oil, plus additional for bread pan
    4–4½ cups whole wheat flour

In a large bowl, dissolve the yeast in the lukewarm water with ½ teaspoon honey. Let sit 10 minutes, until it begins to foam. Stir in the yogurt, remaining honey, the onion, sage, and safflower oil. Beat in the flour, a cup at a time. Use an electric mixer or a wooden spoon. You can knead this dough, which is sticky, in the same fashion that you kneaded the triticale bread (previous recipe), or you can beat it. Beat or knead until thick and elastic (about 10 minutes).

Let the dough rise in the bowl, covered, for 1 to 1½ hours, or until doubled in bulk.

Punch down the dough and turn into an oiled bread pan. Cover and let rise 30 minutes. Toward the end of the rising time, preheat the oven to 350 degrees.

Bake in the preheated oven for 45 minutes, or until the bread is brown and responds to tapping with a hollow thumping sound. Remove from the pan and cool on a rack.

Yeasted Pie Crust

Makes one 10-inch crust

>   1 tablespoon active dry yeast
> 1¼ cups lukewarm water
>   1 teaspoon mild-flavored honey
>   1 tablespoon safflower oil, plus additional
> 3½–4 cups whole wheat flour, as necessary
> corn meal for the pan

In a large bowl, dissolve the yeast in the water with the honey. Let sit 10 minutes, until the yeast foams; then stir in the 1 tablespoon safflower oil and 2 cups of the whole wheat flour, 1 cup at a time. Add another half cup of flour and fold it in. At this point the dough should be a rather sticky mass that can be turned out of the bowl. Place a cup of flour on your kneading surface and turn out the dough. Scrape what remains in the bowl out onto the dough. Flour your hands and begin to knead. Knead, according to the directions on page 177, for about 10 minutes, adding flour as necessary.

Shape the dough into a ball, oil your bowl, and place it in the bowl seam side up first, then seam side down. Cover and let rise in a warm place for 1 to 1½ hours, until doubled in volume. Oil a 10-inch pie pan or baking dish and sprinkle with corn meal.

Punch down and turn out onto a lightly floured kneading surface. Knead a few times, then roll out as thin as possible. Cut away any that you may need for lattice, and line your pie pan or baking dish. At this point the dough can be frozen; it will take only about 15 minutes to thaw.

Prebake for 5 minutes at 400 degrees before filling.

Rye-Oatmeal Bread with Anise and Raisins
Makes 2 loaves

This is an exceptional breakfast bread, but it requires more time than the other two breads here because it is a somewhat heavy dough.

First, mix up half the flour to make a sponge, which rises for an hour. Then, mix in the remaining ingredients and knead. There is an hour-long rise, a 50-minute rise, and another short rise in the pans, all of which makes the recipe take about five hours from start to finish. (Remember, though, you're not working the whole time.) To save time, begin this bread at night and let it rise overnight in the refrigerator. Then it will be piping hot for breakfast.

FOR THE SPONGE

2 tablespoons active dry yeast
3 cups lukewarm water
2 tablespoons molasses
2 cups unbleached white flour
2 cups whole wheat flour

FOR THE REST OF THE BREAD

2 tablespoons safflower oil, plus additional
2 cups rolled oats
2 tablespoons crushed anise seeds
2 tablespoons grated orange rind
1 cup raisins
2 cups rye flour
1 cup whole wheat flour
additional unbleached white flour as necessary, for kneading

Bread

Make the sponge: In a large bowl dissolve the yeast in the lukewarm water and add the molasses. Stir in the 2 cups unbleached flour and the 2 cups whole wheat flour, a cup at a time. (The mixture will resemble thick mud.) Stir it approximately 100 times, cover, and place in warm spot to rise. Let it rise about 60 minutes.

Make the dough: The sponge should now be bubbling. Fold in the 2 tablespoons safflower oil and the oats, a cup at a time, then add the anise seeds, orange rind, and raisins. Fold in the rye flour, a cup at a time. By the time you add your last cup of rye flour, you should be able to turn your dough out of the bowl in a sticky mass. Place a half cup of the whole wheat flour on your kneading surface and turn out the dough. Flour your hands and begin to knead. Knead 10 to 15 minutes, adding more flour as necessary. When you have used up a cup of whole wheat flour and the dough is still sticky, sprinkle the board with unbleached white flour and continue until the dough is smooth and elastic.

Form the dough into a ball, oil your bowl, and place the dough in it seam side up first, then seam side down. Cover and let rise in a warm place for 1 hour.

Punch down the dough and let it rise again, covered, for 50 minutes.

Now turn onto the lightly floured board, knead a few times, and divide into two equal pieces. Form into loaves and place in oiled bread pans, upside down first, then right side up. Let rise 15 to 25 minutes, until the loaves rise above the edges of the pans, while you preheat the oven to 350 degrees.

With a sharp knife, score your loaves 3 times across the top about ½ inch deep. Bake in the preheated oven for 50 minutes, or until the loaves respond to tapping with a hollow thumping sound.

Remove from the pans and cool on a rack.

Yeasted Corn Bread

Serves 12 generously

1 tablespoon active dry yeast
1 cup lukewarm water
2 tablespoons plus ½ teaspoon mild-flavored honey
2 tablespoons flax seeds (available in health food stores)
1 cup Homemade Nonfat Yogurt (page 217)
3 tablespoons safflower oil, plus additional for baking dish
3 cups stone-ground yellow corn meal
1 cup whole wheat pastry flour

Dissolve the yeast in ½ cup warm water with ½ teaspoon honey. Let sit for 10 minutes, until it begins to foam.

Meanwhile, grind up the flax seeds in a blender or spice mill. Place in a bowl and pour in the other ½ cup warm water. The flax seeds will become viscous and will act like egg whites in the batter.

Combine the yogurt, 2 tablespoons honey, and 3 tablespoons safflower oil. When the yeast has begun to foam, stir the yogurt mixture and blend in the flax seeds.

Sift together the corn meal and whole wheat pastry flour. Stir in the wet ingredients with just a few strokes. The batter should be lumpy.

Pour into an oiled 2- or 3-quart baking dish and set aside to rise for 30 minutes. Meanwhile, preheat the oven to 375 degrees. Bake in the preheated oven for 40 minutes until the bread begins to brown on top. Cool in the pan or serve hot.

Whole Grain Croutons

Croutons given an added crunchy texture to salads and impart a wholesome flavor. These dry croutons can be made from any whole grain bread that is beginning to dry out.

Slice up to 1 loaf of bread and dice the slices into small pieces. Preheat the oven to 300 degrees. Place the bread in an ungreased baking dish and bake for 30 minutes. Remove from the oven and allow to cool.

Herbed Bread Crumbs
Makes 3 cups

These make a nice topping for casseroles and a tasty addition to salads. They can be stored for a week or so in the refrigerator or they can be frozen.

    1 teaspoon safflower oil
    2 large cloves garlic
    2 cups whole wheat bread crumbs
    ½ cup finely chopped fresh parsley
    2 teaspoons grated lemon peel
    freshly ground pepper to taste

Heat the oil in a heavy-bottomed skillet and add the garlic. Cook a few seconds, then add the bread crumbs. Cook, stirring, until they begin to toast and dry, about 5 minutes. Stir in the remaining ingredients and sauté another 2 minutes or so. Remove from the heat.

Note: Bread crumbs can be made in a blender or food processor. Cut slices of bread into quarters and run at high speed until uniform. In general, 2 slices of bread will yield ½ cup bread crumbs.

Corn Tortillas

If you can't find good bread without salt, and don't want to make your own, packaged corn tortillas will make a good staple. Many brands contain no salt. They go beautifully with beans, vegetables, and grains. To heat tortillas, either place on a steamer over boiling water and steam them for a minute or so, heat in a dry pan on both sides above a medium flame, or wrap in foil and place in the oven. If you want chips, you can cut the tortillas into wedges and bake them for 15 minutes in a preheated 250-degree oven.

Soft tacos can be served the traditional way—with beans and salsa. Or try them with leftover vegetables or casseroles. Just heat a tortilla, fill it with beans or vegetables, top with sprouts or shredded lettuce, and season with Salsa Fresca (see page 205).

Crackers

Check the packages carefully. Look for brands that contain no added salt, sugar, or fats, such as Kavli, Ideal, Ry-Krisp, and various eggless matzohs.

17. Spreads and Pâtés

Bean spreads are economical and easy to make. When eaten with whole grain breads, they form a complete protein. Leftover vegetable dishes, beans, or casseroles can be seasoned with lemon juice, garlic, pepper, or herbs, puréed, refrigerated, and used as sandwich spreads for the rest of the week. Other seasonings that can be tried with leftover beans are paprika, thyme, cardamom, cayenne, or chili pepper. The White Bean Spread (see below) is a good model recipe for using leftover beans, and the Spinach Yogurt Spread (see page 190) can be used as a model for using leftover vegetables. Try adding a little garlic or your own favorite herbs.

Most of these recipes can be frozen and kept for several days. (Recipes that include tofu as an ingredient are best not frozen, since the texture of tofu is considerably altered by freezing.)

White Bean Spread

Makes 3 cups

White beans have a sutble flavor, are extremely versatile, and make a surprisingly delicous pâté.

  1 cup white beans, washed, picked over, and soaked
  1 small onion, chopped
  5 cloves garlic, minced or put through a press
  1 bay leaf
  2 sprigs parsley
  ¼ teaspoon dried thyme

3 cups water
juice of 1 lemon (or more, to taste)
2 tablespoons sesame tahini
freshly ground pepper to taste
1 teaspoon ground cumin (optional)
½ teaspoon ground coriander (optional)
2–3 tablespoons red wine vinegar, to taste (optional)
1 or more teaspoons prepared mustard, to taste (optional)

Combine the beans, onion, 3 cloves of the garlic, the bay leaf, parsley, thyme, and water in a saucepan and bring to a boil. Cover, reduce heat, and simmer 1½ hours, or until tender. Drain the beans and remove the bay leaf and parsley.

Blend in a blender or food processor with the remaining garlic and other ingredients until smooth. Transfer to a covered jar and chill.

Garbanzo or Black-eyed Pea Spread
Makes 3 cups

Substitute black-eyed peas or garbanzos for the white beans and proceed as in the recipe above.

White Bean Pesto Spread
Makes 2½ cups

If you love sweet basil and have access to it, you will likely enjoy this spread. It's like eating pesto Genovese, the traditionally high-fat basil sauce, without the olive oil or Parmesan. You still get the garlic, basil, and the subtle background of the white beans. (If you have less time, you can cook the white beans more simply, as on page 171.)

3 cups water
¾ cup white beans, washed, picked over, and soaked
½ onion, chopped
4 large cloves garlic, minced or put through a press
1 bay leaf
1 sprig parsley
1 cup, tightly packed, fresh basil leaves
juice of 1 lemon
2 tablespoons sesame tahini
freshly ground pepper

Combine the water, beans, onion, 2 cloves of the garlic, the bay leaf, and the parsley in a saucepan and bring to a boil. Cover, reduce heat, and cook 1½ hours, or until the beans are tender. Drain. Discard bay leaf.

Chop the basil with the remaining garlic very fine in a blender or food processor. Add the beans, lemon juice, and tahini and blend until smooth. Season with pepper to taste. Transfer to a covered container and chill.

Mushroom Spread
Makes 2½ cups

    1 teaspoon safflower oil
    3 cloves garlic, minced or put through a press
    1 pound mushrooms, wiped clean, stems trimmed
    3 green onions, sliced
    3 tablespoons dry white wine
    ½ teaspoon dried thyme
    2 tablespoons lemon juice
    1 teaspoon grated lemon rind
    freshly ground pepper to taste
    ¼ cup chopped fresh parsley (optional)

Heat the safflower oil in a large, heavy-bottomed skillet and add the garlic. Sauté 1 minute, and add the mushrooms and green onions. Sauté, stirring, for a minute, then add the wine and the thyme. Cook over a medium flame, stirring, for about 10 minutes, or until the liquid evaporates and the mushrooms are tender and aromatic.

Remove from the heat and purée in a food processor, through a food mill, or in a blender. Season to taste with lemon juice, lemon rind, freshly ground pepper, and, if you wish, fresh parsley. Chill in a covered container.

Curried Lentil and Apple Spread
Makes 3 cups

The pungent flavor of the curry and cumin makes an interesting contrast with the tart apples. If you don't like curried foods, try this without the spices—lentils have so much character of their own that it will still be tasy.

This recipe will keep for several days in the refrigerator, and it freezes well.

1 cup lentils, washed and picked over
½ onion, minced.
2 large cloves garlic, minced or put through a press
1 bay leaf
1 teaspoon ground cumin
2 teaspoons curry powder
½ cup raw brown rice, washed
4 cups water
2 tart apples, such as Granny Smith, peeled, grated, or
   minced and tossed with the juice of ½ lemon
lots of freshly ground pepper
1–2 teaspoons Homemade Mustard Without Salt (page 211)
   (optional)

Combine the lentils, onion, garlic, bay leaf, cumin, curry powder, brown rice, and water in a saucepan and bring to a boil. Reduce heat, cover, and simmer 45 minutes, until the rice and lentils are tender. Drain, retaining the liquid if you wish, for another use. Remove the bay leaf.

Blend the mixture in a blender or food processor until smooth. Stir in the apples, pepper, and mustard. Transfer to a covered jar and chill. Serve on bread.

Eggplant Caviar

Makes 3 cups

1½ pounds eggplant
2 teaspoons safflower oil
½ onion, sliced thin
2 cloves garlic, minced or put through a press
1 large red or green pepper, minced
3 tomatoes, peeled (see Note) and chopped
2 tablespoons unsalted tomato paste
1 teaspoon mild-flavored honey
¼ cup vinegar
freshly ground pepper to taste
allspice to taste
lemon juice to taste (optional)
strips of lemon zest from 1 lemon
½ green pepper, cut in lengthwise strips
½ red pepper, cut in lengthwise strips

Preheat oven to 450 degrees. Pierce the eggplant in several places with a knife or skewer and bake for 20 to 30 minutes, or until soft. Remove from the heat and when cool enough to handle, cut in half, scoop out the pulp, and chop.

Heat the safflower oil and sauté the onion with the garlic until tender. Add the minced green pepper, tomatoes, tomato paste, eggplant, honey, and vinegar and cook together for about 10 minutes, stirring occasionally. Remove from the heat and season to taste with freshly ground pepper, allspice, and if you wish, lemon juice.

Transfer to a serving dish and garnish with strips of lemon zest (the yellow part of the peel) and green and red peppers. Cover and chill.

Note: To peel tomatoes, drop into boiling water for 20 seconds, drain, and run under cold water.

Spinach Yogurt Spread
Makes 1½ cups

This recipe is very easy, and can be used interchangeably as a dip or a spread.

    10 ounces frozen spinach, thawed
    juice of ½ lemon
    ¼ cup Homemade Nonfat Yogurt (page 217)

Wrap the thawed spinach in a towel and squeeze out all the liquid. Purée in a blender or food processor with the lemon juice and yogurt. Chill in a covered container.

Bean Mustard Mayonnaise
Makes 1¼ cups

This tart spread can be spread on bread or used as a dip in much the same way as you would use mayonnaise.

    1 cup cooked white beans (pages 171–172)
    3 tablespoons vinegar
    1 tablespoon Homemade Mustard Without Salt (page 211)
    1 clove garlic (optional)
    freshly ground pepper to taste
    lemon juice to taste

Blend all the ingredients together in a blender or food processor until smooth. Thin with more vinegar if you wish.

Black Bean Dip

Makes 3 cups

    1 cup black beans, washed, picked over and soaked
    1 onion, chopped
    3 cloves garlic, minced or put through a press
    3 cups water
    1 jalapeño, seeds removed, cut in strips
    1 tablespoon chopped fresh coriander (cilantro)
    2 teaspoons ground cumin (more to taste)
    2 teaspoons chili powder (more to taste)
    2 tablespoons red wine vinegar (optional)

Combine the beans, onion, garlic, water, jalapeño, and coriander (cilantro) in a bean pot and bring to a boil. Reduce heat, cover, and cook 1½ to 2 hours, until the beans are tender. Drain.

Purée in a blender or food processor with the remaining ingredients. Do not purée until completely smooth, but leave a little texture. Adjust seasonings.

Note: Black Bean Dip is a natural to serve with nachos. To make nachos, cut corn tortillas into pie-shaped wedges. Preheat the oven to 250 degrees and place the tortilla wedges on baking sheets. Bake 20 minutes, or until crisp but not brown. Serve with the black beans, with Salsa Fresca (see page 205) or more jalapeños.

Herbed Tofu Spread

Makes 1½ cups

    ½ pound tofu
    3–4 tablespoons vinegar or lemon juice, or a combination
    2 teaspoons Homemade Mustard Without Salt (page 211)
    3–4 tablespoons fresh chopped herbs, such as basil, parsley,
       dill, thyme, tarragon, marjoram, rosemary
    freshly ground pepper to taste
    1 large or 2 small tomatoes, puréed
    1 small bell pepper, minced

Mash the tofu with a fork and mix in the other ingredients. Chill in a covered container. Serve on bread, or eat like cottage cheese.

Apple Spice Tofu Morning Special

Makes 2 cups

If you don't like tofu because you think of it as bland and uninteresting, this spread should be a pleasant surprise. It is sweet, creamy, and almost like cheesecake when served on toast.

safflower oil for baking dish.
2 medium-size tart apples or ⅔ cup unsweetened applesauce
½ pound (2 cakes) tofu
¼ cup Homemade Nonfat Yogurt (page 217)
1–2 tablespoons mild-flavored honey, maple syrup, or sorghum syrup
1–2 tablespoons lemon juice
½ teaspoon cinnamon
½ teaspoon nutmeg
1 tablespoon sesame tahini
1 teaspoon vanilla extract
2 teaspoons whole wheat pastry flour

Preheat the oven to 350 degrees. If you are using whole apples, oil a small baking dish or a 1-quart casserole. Bake the apples for 30 to 45 minutes, until thoroughly soft. Remove from the heat and core when cool enough to handle.

Blend all the ingredients together, including the apples or applesauce, skins and all, until very smooth. Pour into the oiled baking dish. Bake 30 to 40 minutes, until firm and just beginning to brown. Cool and refrigerate in a covered container.

Peanut Butter Banana Tofu Spread

Makes 2 cups

safflower oil for baking dish
½ pound (2 cakes) tofu
¼ cup Homemade Nonfat Yogurt (page 217)
2 tablespoons mild-flavored honey
1 large banana or 2 small bananas
2 tablespoons unsalted peanut butter
½ teaspoon cinnamon
½ teaspoon nutmeg
1 teaspoon vanilla extract
1 tablespoon lemon juice
2 teaspoons whole wheat pastry flour

Preheat the oven to 350 degrees. Lightly oil a small baking dish or a 1-quart casserole.

Blend all the ingredients together until smooth. Pour into the baking dish and bake 30 to 40 minutes, until firm and just beginning to brown. Remove from the oven, cool, and chill. Will keep 1 week.

Apricot Preserves

Makes 1½ pints

> ¾ pound pitted dried apricots
> 2½ cups water
> ½ teaspoon almond extract
> juice and grated rind of 1 orange (optional)

Place the apricots in a bowl and cover with the water. Soak overnight. When thoroughly softened, purée in a blender or food processor. Add the almond extract, orange juice, and rind (if you wish).

Transfer to a stainless or enamel saucepan and simmer over low heat for 15 to 30 minutes, until thick. Cool and store in the refrigerator in covered jars.

18. Dressings and Sauces

The word "sauce" conjures up visions of rich butter sauce and hollandaise, and "dressings" are usually synonymous with oil. But butter is not the only thing that will melt in your mouth, and an oil vinaigrette is not the only kind of dressing that enhances a salad. There are many kinds of low-fat, salt-free toppings that will liven up vegetables, grains, and pasta.

The traditional way of thickening sauces has been either with a combination of butter and flour or with an emulsion of oil and eggs. Yet there are many other ways to make a thick sauce. Arrowroot and cornstarch will thicken simmering liquids to make smooth, silky adornments for vegetables, grains, and pasta; puréed vegetables like mushrooms and tomatoes will provide a large number of savory possibilities. Think of the smooth, light, and delicious sauces surrounding many of the entrées from Oriental and Chinese kitchens—these are usually based on cornstarch rather than butter.

Most commercial salad dressings are high in both calories and fat. But salad dressings need not pose a problem. The following pages contain recipes for sixteen low-fat, low-salt, low-calorie dressings. Some are sweet and fruity, others are sour, a few are spicy—and all are tasty. They can be enjoyed over vegetables, grains, and pasta as well as salads. These dressings can help to transform a simple meal into a fancy one.

The recipes here are just a starting point. As you become familiar with the underlying concepts, you may want to experiment with other foods and develop your own dressings.

Low-Fat Vinaigrette
Makes 1 cup

Though this is a much thinner version of its oily counterpart, it will stick to the salad greens. A little bit of oil goes a long way. This will hold up to 5 days in the refrigerator, but it is best served fresh. It deteriorates in flavor if frozen.

> juice of ½ lemon
> 3–4 tablespoons wine or cider vinegar
> 1 clove garlic, minced or put through a press
> ½ teaspoon dry mustard or 1 teaspoon Homemade Mustard
>   Without Salt (page 211)
> ¼ teaspoon dried marjoram or basil
> ¼ teaspoon dried tarragon
> 2–3 teaspoons fresh chopped herbs, if available, such as
>   basil, thyme, dill, fennel, marjoram, parsley, chives
> freshly ground pepper to taste
> 2 tablespoons safflower oil
> ½ cup water

Blend all the ingredients together in a blender or food processor for about 30 seconds. Shake before using.

Yogurt Vinaigrette
Makes 1 cup

This is a creamy version of the low-fat vinaigrette. It will hold for about 5 days in the refrigerator, but it does not freeze.

> juice of ½ lemon
> 3 tablespoons wine vinegar
> 1 clove garlic, minced or put through a press
> ½ teaspoon dry mustard or 1 teaspoon Homemade Mustard
>   Without Salt (page 211)
> ¼ teaspoon dried marjoram or basil
> ¼ teaspoon dried tarragon
> 2 teaspoons chopped fresh dill or 1 teaspoon dried
> freshly ground pepper to taste
> ½–¾ cup Homemade Nonfat Yogurt (page 217)

Mix together all the ingredients except the yogurt. Combine well and whisk in the yogurt. Chill until ready to use.

Tomato Vinaigrette
Makes 1 cup

Same ingredients as Yogurt Vinaigrette (above), but substitute 1 large, ripe tomato for the yogurt. Liquefy all the ingredients in a blender and add seasonings. You might want to add fresh herbs such as basil, oregano, or thyme (1 to 3 teaspoons each).

Parsley Vinaigrette
Makes 1 cup

Add ½ cup chopped fresh parsley to the basic Low-Fat Vinaigrette recipe and blend together in a blender until smooth.

Curried Vinaigrette
Makes 1 cup

Add 1 teaspoon curry powder to the basic Low-Fat Vinaigrette recipe and stir well.

Basil or Dill Vinaigrette
Makes 1–1½ cups

Add ¼ to ½ cup fresh basil or fresh dill and another clove of garlic to the Tomato Vinaigrette and blend until smooth.

White Bean Vinaigrette
Makes 1½ cups

Substitute ½ cup cooked white beans for the water in the basic Low-Fat Vinaigrette; blend until smooth. Thin to desired consistency with water, lemon juice, or liquid from the beans. Add additional lemon juice as desired.

Garbanzo Vinaigrette
Makes 1½ cups

Substitute ½ cup cooked garbanzos for the water in the basic Low-Fat Vinaigrette and 1 tablespoon sesame tahini for 1 tablespoon of the safflower oil. Add additional garlic if you wish, and blend until smooth. Thin with water, lemon juice, or liquid from the beans. Add additional lemon juice as desired.

Poppy Seed Dressing
Makes 1½ cups

⅓ cup lemon juice
2 tablespoons mild-flavored honey
2 tablespoons cider vinegar
2 tablespoons poppy seeds
¾ cup Homemade Nonfat Yogurt (page 217)

Stir together all the ingredients except the yogurt. Make sure the honey is dissolved, then stir in the yogurt.

Green Gazpacho Dressing
Makes 2 cups

If you get tired of putting this tart, vitamin-rich dressing on salads, try eating it as a soup. This will hold for up to a week in the refrigerator, though the fresher it is the better it tastes. It does not freeze.

2 tablespoons coarsely chopped onion
1 clove garlic, peeled
½ bell pepper, seeds removed, cut in half or quarters
1 tablespoon chopped fresh basil
2 sprigs parsley
¼ teaspoon dried tarragon
¼–½ teaspoon dried marjoram, to taste
1½ cups quartered ripe tomatoes
juice of 1 large lemon
2 tablespoons vinegar
freshly ground pepper to taste
2 tablespoons safflower oil or Homemade Nonfat Yogurt (page 217) (optional)

Purée all the ingredients in a blender until smooth. Chill until ready to serve.

Hot and Sour Dressing
Makes 1½ cups

>   3 tablespoons sesame tahini
>   4 tablespoons cider or white wine vinegar
>   1 teaspoon hot red pepper powder or flaked red pepper
>   2 tablespoons lemon juice
>   1 teaspoon mild-flavored honey
>   1 tablespoon finely minced or grated fresh ginger
>   1–2 cloves garlic, finely minced
>   1 tablespoon finely minced scallions
>   1 tablespoon safflower oil
>   1 tablespoon chopped fresh coriander (cilantro) (optional)
>   ½ cup water
>   freshly ground pepper to taste

In a blender or food processor, blend all the ingredients together until smooth. Refrigerate until ready to use. Shake before tossing with the salad.

Tri-Sprout Dressing
Makes 1½ cups

This is one of the many creations of Connie Colten, who was an assistant cook during the program.

>   1 tablespoon chopped onion
>   ¼ cup lentil sprouts
>   ¼ cup mung bean sprouts
>   ¼ cup alfalfa sprouts
>   juice of 1 lemon
>   ¼ cup cider vinegar
>   1 tablespoon sesame tahini
>   1 teaspoon paprika
>   1 teaspoon grated fresh ginger
>   1 tomato
>   freshly ground pepper to taste

Blend all the ingredients together until smooth. Store in the refrigerator.

Orange-Peach Dressing
Makes 1½ cups

>3 dried apricots
>juice of 1 lemon
>juice of 1 orange
>1 large or 2 small ripe peaches, peeled, stones removed
>¼–½ teaspoon dry mustard, to taste
>¼ teaspoon cinnamon
>½ cup Homemade Nonfat Yogurt (page 217)

Place the apricots in a bowl and pour on boiling water to cover. Let sit 10 minutes and drain.

Blend all the ingredients (including the apricots) until smooth in a blender or food processor. Refrigerate until ready to use.

Pineapple Sesame Dressing
Makes 1 cup

>⅔ cup fresh chopped pineapple
>2 tablespoons wine or cider vinegar
>2 tablespoons lemon or lime juice
>2 tablespoon sesame tahini

Purée all the ingredients in a blender or food processor until smooth. Refrigerate until ready to use.

Fresh Coriander Dressing
Makes 1¼ cups

Another contribution from Connie Colten.

¼ cup chopped fresh coriander (cilantro)
1 teaspoon ground coriander seed
½ teaspoon curry powder
¼ teaspoon anise seeds
¼ cup vinegar
juice of 1 lime
¼ cup alfalfa sprouts
1 tablespoon safflower oil
1 tablespoon Homemade Nonfat Yogurt (page 217)
1 teaspoon chopped onion
1 tomato

Blend all the ingredients together until smooth.

Simple Tomato Sauce

Makes 3½ cups

This sauce goes well with grains and steamed vegetables as well as with pasta. It can be stored for up to a week in the refrigerator, and it freezes well.

2 teaspoons safflower oil
1 small onion, finely chopped
2 cloves garlic, minced or put through a press
3 pounds ripe tomatoes, seeded and puréed, or 3 pounds canned tomatoes, seeded and puréed
freshly ground pepper to taste
pinch of cinnamon
1–2 teaspoons fresh basil or ½ teaspoon dried or more to taste (optional)
½–1 teaspoon dried oregano (optional)
¼ teaspoon dried thyme (optional)

Heat the oil in a heavy-bottomed saucepan, large frying pan, or Dutch oven and sauté the onion and garlic gently until the onion is translucent. Add the tomatoes, stir, and simmer gently, uncovered, for 20 minutes. Add freshly ground pepper, a pinch of cinnamon, and the optional herbs. Simmer a little longer if you wish, and remove from the heat.

Picante Tomato Sauce

Makes 5 cups

> 3½ pounds tomatoes, fresh or canned
> 2 teaspoons safflower oil
> 2 large cloves garlic, minced or put through a press
> 3 tablespoons chopped fresh basil or 1 tablespoon dried
> 1 teaspoon crushed dried red pepper (you can do this in a spice mill or chop it finely with a sharp knife)

Purée the tomatoes coarsely in a food processor, blender, or through a food mill.

Heat the oil in a large, heavy-bottomed saucepan or skillet and sauté the garlic gently until it begins to color, about 1 to 2 minutes. Add the tomatoes, basil, and hot red pepper and bring to a simmer, stirring. Cook uncovered over moderate heat, stirring occasionally, for 20 to 30 minutes, until the sauce thickens.

"Gravy"

Makes 3 cups

You can make gravy or sauces from many things. The best ingredients are soups and beans, which you can blend and season with tomatoes, vinegar, or spices.

If you don't have anything cooked on hand to blend, try the recipe below:

> 2 pounds tomatoes
> 1 onion, coarsely chopped
> 1 tablespoon mild-flavored honey
> 3 tablespoons vinegar (more to taste)
> 3 cloves garlic
> 1 tablespoon whole wheat flour
> freshly ground pepper

Combine everything except the whole wheat flour and pepper together in a blender until smooth.

Heat the flour in a dry skillet and when it begins to brown, whisk in the tomato purée. Cook, stirring, for 10 minutes. Add freshly ground pepper to taste.

Sweet Yogurt Cereal Topping
Makes 2 cups

Even if you don't like yogurt you might like this, because the banana and apple juice sweeten it and add flavor.

    1 cup Homemade Nonfat Yogurt (page 217)
    ¼ cup unfiltered apple juice
    ½ ripe banana
    ¼ cup water
    ½ teaspoon vanilla extract

Blend all the ingredients together until smooth. Refrigerate until ready to use.

Mushroom Sauce
Makes 1½ cups

This is a savory, velvety sauce, with all the attributes of a thick mushroom soup, but without the cream or butter. It will keep up to 3 days in the refrigerator, in a covered container, and freezes well. Substitute it for mushroom gravy on potatoes, or serve it over vegetables or grains.

    2 teaspoons safflower oil
    ½ medium onion, minced, or 3 shallots, minced
    ½ pound mushrooms, wiped, stems trimmed, and sliced
    1 large clove garlic or 2 smaller cloves, crushed or minced
    ¼ cup dry white wine
    ¼ teaspoon dried thyme
    pinch of nutmeg
    1½ cups water
    freshly ground pepper
    1 tablespoon dry sherry

Heat the oil in a heavy-bottomed, 2- or 3-quart saucepan (or you can use a larger pan, such as a Dutch oven or soup pot). Sauté the onion until tender, about 3 to 5 minutes. Add the mushrooms and garlic and sauté over medium heat for about 5 minutes, stirring, or until the liquid evaporates. Add the wine, thyme, and nutmeg and turn up the heat. Cook, stirring, until the wine has just about evaporated, and pour in the water. Bring to a simmer, cover, and reduce heat. Cook 15 minutes.

Drain the mushrooms and retain the liquid. Purée with 1 cup of the cooking liquid in a blender, until completely smooth. (A blender is better than a food processor for this, because the food processor leaves little chunks.) Thin out to the desired consistency with the remaining cooking liquid and season to taste with freshly ground pepper. Stir in the sherry, heat through, and serve.

Puréed Eggplant Sauce
Makes 1½ cups

When baked at high heat, the eggplant becomes pungent and the purée, seasoned with garlic and lemon juice, will be smooth and silky. You can make a textured sauce by adding any of the variations below. Experiment with seasonings. This will keep up to 5 days in the refrigerator.

    1 teaspoon safflower oil, for the baking sheet
    1 medium-size eggplant (approximately 1 pound)
    2 cloves garlic
    3 tablespoons lemon juice
    freshly ground pepper to taste
    ½ cup Homemade Nonfat Yogurt (page 217)
    2 tablespoons chopped parsley, or 1 tablespoon parsley and
      1 tablespoon chopped fresh basil

Preheat the oven to 500 degrees. Oil a baking sheet. Cut the eggplant in half lengthwise and score each half twice, down to the skin but not through it. Lay the eggplants cut side down on the baking sheet and bake for 20 minutes. Remove from the heat and allow to cool.

When the eggplant is cool enough to handle, scoop out the pulp and transfer to a blender jar or food processor. Purée with the garlic, lemon juice, freshly ground pepper, and yogurt until completely smooth. Stir in the parsley and basil. Reheat gently.

Puréed Eggplant Sauce with Fresh Coriander

Makes 2 cups

Stir into the Puréed Eggplant Sauce any or all of the following: 2 tablespoons chopped fresh coriander (cilantro), ½ cup minced bell pepper, and 1 ripe tomato, peeled and chopped.

Curried Eggplant Sauce

Makes 1½ cups

Add 1 to 2 teaspoons curry powder to the Puréed Eggplant Sauce recipe and stir well.

Puréed Eggplant Sauce with Cumin

Makes 1½ cups

Add ½ teaspoon cumin, or more to taste, to the Puréed Eggplant Sauce recipe and stir well.

Lemon-Ginger Sauce

Makes ⅔ cup

> ¼ cup fresh lemon juice
> 1 teaspoon grated fresh ginger
> 2 teaspoons mild-flavored honey
> ⅓ cup plus 1 tablespoon water
> 2 teaspoons cornstarch
> 2 teaspoons dry sherry

Combine the lemon juice, ginger, honey, and ⅓ cup water in a saucepan. Heat to a simmer.

Dissolve the cornstarch in the additional tablespoon of water and stir into the lemon juice mixture. Simmer, stirring, until the mixture thickens. Stir in the sherry. Serve with vegetables or grains.

Creamy Garlic Sauce

Makes 1 cup

Don't be alarmed by all the garlic used in this. As it simmers, it loses its harsh flavor. This sauce goes well with mashed potatoes, cauliflower, and green vegetables. It can be frozen and will keep for 3 days in the refrigerator.

15 cloves garlic, peeled and left whole
1½ cups water
pinch of dried sage
pinch of dried thyme
juice of ½ lemon (more to taste)
2 tablespoons dry white wine
2 tablespoons chopped fresh parsley
freshly ground pepper

Combine the garlic, water, sage, and thyme in a saucepan and simmer uncovered for 30 to 40 minutes. Remove from the heat and purée in a blender until smooth. Add the lemon juice and white wine. Return to the saucepan and stir in the parsley and freshly ground pepper to taste. Heat thoroughly over very low heat.

Salsa Fresca

Makes 1½ cups

This uncooked pincante sauce can add a Mexican flair to any meal, whether or not you have tortillas to go with it. The fresh coriander leaves makes this special. The salsa is best if served fresh, but will hold up to 3 days in the refrigerator, in a covered container. It does not freeze.

3 medium-size ripe tomatoes (1 pound), minced
½ small onion, minced
6 sprigs fresh coriander (cilantro), minced
2 serrano or jalapeño chilies, minced
¼ cup red wine vinegar
⅓ cup water

Combine all the minced vegetables with the vinegar and water. Serve at once, or chill and serve.

White Wine Sauce
Makes 1 cup

This is an elegant sauce. Dried mushrooms and garlic are simmered in white wine, and the heady liquid that results is thickened (after the mushrooms and garlic are removed) with arrowroot or cornstarch. It's as simple as that. Serve on grain dishes or vegetables. It will stay fresh for up to 3 days in the refrigerator, but it does not freeze well.

    6 dried Chinese mushrooms
    6 cloves garlic, peeled and left whole
    1 cup dry white wine
    ½ cup water
    4 teaspoons cornstarch or arrowroot
    freshly ground pepper to taste

Combine the Chinese mushrooms, garlic, wine, and water in a saucepan and simmer, covered, for 30 to 40 minutes. Strain and return the liquid to the saucepan. Hold the mushrooms for optional use in the sauce or for use in another vegetable dish (they are too precious to throw away).

Spoon 2 tablespoons of the broth into a small dish and dissolve the cornstarch or arrowroot in it. Place the remaining broth over a medium-high flame and stir in the dissolved cornstarch or arrowroot. Stir until the mixture comes to a boil and thickens. Add pepper to taste. It will not be much thicker than a glaze at first, but you can reduce it to the desired consistency. If you wish, mince the reserved mushrooms and add to the sauce.

Low-Fat Tomato "Béarnaise"
Makes 1 cup

This sauce can be called a béarnaise because of the reduction in vinegar, but it has little else in common with the traditional sauce, which is based on butter and eggs. The tart, savory flavor of this sauce goes well with vegetables. It will freeze well and can be refrigerated for up to 4 days.

4 tablespoons red wine vinegar
⅓ cup minced shallots or white part of green onion
3 tablespoons minced carrot
2 large ripe tomatoes, peeled (see Note), seeded, and chopped
2 tablespoons chopped fresh parsley
¼ teaspoon tarragon
½ cup water
1 tablespoon safflower oil
freshly ground pepper
1–2 teaspoons chopped fresh herbs such as basil, parsley, thyme, dill (optional)

Combine the vinegar, shallots or green onions, and carrot in a small heavy-bottomed saucepan and place over moderate heat. Simmer the mixture until almost all of the vinegar has evaporated. There should be only enough left so that the vegetables aren't completely dry. Add the chopped tomatoes and continue to cook, stirring occasionally, for about 15 minutes, until the mixture is almost dry again. About 5 minutes before the end of this cooking, stir in the parsley and tarragon.

Remove from the heat and transfer to a blender. Blend, along with the water, until smooth. While the blender is running, drizzle in the oil.

Transfer the puréed sauce back to the saucepan, season to taste with pepper, and if you wish, add chopped fresh herbs. Heat through gently and serve. Alternatively, serve cold.

Note: To peel tomatoes, drop into boiling water for 20 seconds, drain, and run under cold water.

Curried Cauliflower-Yogurt Sauce
Makes 1¼ cups

This goes well with vegetables and potatoes. It will last 3 days in the refrigerator and can be frozen.

¼ pound chopped cauliflower
2 teaspoons chopped onion
½–1 teaspoon curry powder
¼–½ teaspoon ground cumin, to taste
freshly ground pepper to taste
½ cup Homemade Nonfat Yogurt (page 217), or more to taste

Steam the cauliflower for 10 to 15 minutes, until tender. Drain and purée with the onion, curry powder, cumin, pepper, and yogurt in a blender or food processor. Adjust seasoning, and if you want a thinner sauce, add more yogurt. Heat through over low heat, being careful not to boil or the yogurt will curdle.

Special Strawberry Sauce
Makes 1 cup

The raspberry vinegar and the cardamom make this special. An elegant topping for fruits or yogurt, it will hold 4 days in the refrigerator but should not be frozen.

> 1 cup strawberries, hulled and quartered
> ¼ cup water
> ¼ cup dry white wine
> 2 tablespoons raspberry vinegar (available in specialty food stores)
> 1 tablespoon mild-flavored honey
> ⅛ teaspoon ground cardamom
> 1½ teaspoons cornstarch dissolved in 1 tablespoon water

Combine the strawberries, water, white wine, vinegar, and honey in a heavy-bottomed saucepan and bring to a simmer. Simmer 5 minutes and stir in the cardamom and the dissolved cornstarch. Cook, stirring, another 5 minutes and remove from the heat. Serve hot or at room temperature.

Plum Sauce
Makes 2 cups

> 2 pounds ripe red plums, pitted and sliced
> 1 cup water
> ¼ cup mild-flavored honey
> 1 tablespoon arrowroot or cornstarch dissolved in 2 tablespoons water (optional)

Combine the plums and water in a saucepan and bring to a boil. Reduce heat and simmer 3 minutes. Add the honey, stir well, and remove from the heat. Cover and let sit overnight.

The next day, bring the mixture to a simmer again and cook, stirring, until the mixture thickens. This should take about 30 minutes. You can also thicken the sauce by stirring in the arrowroot or cornstarch dissolved in water. Stir until thick and remove from the heat. Keep refrigerated in covered jars.

19. Mustards and Relishes

Dill pickles are loaded with salt, but many other condiments such as mustards, catsup, tomato relish, and chutneys can be made without it. They may taste different from the commercial brands you are used to, but the important elements are there. Mustard, for instance, is based mainly on mustard seeds and vinegar, and here we have three variations on that theme. Catsup and tomato relish are based on tomatoes, spices, and vinegar.

Fruit and vegetable chutneys make nice condiments for grain and vegetable dishes, especially curries. A little goes a long way, so if you make up a batch you will have it on hand for a long time. Pungent and spicy, chutneys will add flavor to any dish.

Another item in the "condiment" category is vinegar. This may become one of your primary seasonings. There is an amazing array of vinegars now available, in addition to the familiar red and white wine, cider, and distilled varieties. Champagne vinegar has a delicious flavor, and Italian balsamic vinegar is almost sweet at the same time that it is sour. There are also several flavored types—herbal vinegars like garlic, thyme, basil, tarragon, and mint, hot pepper infusions, and sweet varieties like raspberry and strawberry. These are all available in gourmet food shops and in some supermarkets. You can also make your own, by adding various ingredients to regular vinegar. For recipes, see *Better Than Store-Bought*, by Helen Witty and Elizabeth Schneider Colchie (Harper & Row, 1979).

HOMEMADE MUSTARDS WITHOUT SALT

Instead of buying those expensive varieties from France and England, you can make your own mustard in minutes and at a fraction of the cost. It is amazingly easy. The distinctive flavor of mustard is a combination of vinegar and other pungent seasonings with the sharply flavored mustard seed. Homemade mustard also makes a nice holiday gift.

Coarse-Ground Mustard with Red Wine and Garlic
Makes about 1 cup

> ¼ cup mustard seeds
> 2 tablespoons red wine
> ⅓ cup red wine vinegar
> ¼ cup water
> ¼ teaspoon ground allspice
> ½ teaspoon mild-flavored honey
> ¼ teaspoon freshly ground pepper
> ½–1 teaspoon minced garlic, to taste
> 1 small bay leaf, finely crumbled or ground

Combine the mustard seeds, red wine, and vinegar in a dish and let stand for 3 hours or more.

Put the mixture into a blender jar or food processor and add the remaining ingredients. Purée to a coarse texture.

Scrape into the top of a double boiler and stir over simmering water for 5 to 10 minutes, until the mixture has thickened somewhat. Scrape into a jar, cool, and refrigerate.

Green Peppercorn Mustard
Makes about 1½ cups

This is an extra-hot mustard.

3 tablespoons mustard seeds
⅓ cup ground dry mustard
½ cup hot tap water
½ cup white wine vinegar
¼ cup dry white wine or dry white vermouth
¼ teaspoon ground cinnamon
½ teaspoon dried tarragon, crumbled
½ teaspoon dill seeds
large pinch of ground cloves
1 teaspoon mild-flavored honey
1 tablespoon freeze-dried green peppercorns

Combine the mustard seeds, dry mustard, water, and vinegar in a bowl and let stand for at least 3 hours.

Combine the wine or vermouth, cinnamon, tarragon, dill seeds, and cloves in a small saucepan and bring to a boil. Strain into the mustard mixture and stir. Add the honey and green peppercorns.

Scrape into a food processor or blender and purée. Transfer to the top of a double boiler and cook over simmering water for 10 minutes, stirring often. Scrape into a jar, cool, and refrigerate.

Tarragon Mustard
Makes about 1 cup

¼ cup mustard seeds
2 tablespoons dry white wine or dry white vermouth
⅓ cup white wine vinegar
2 teaspoons dried tarragon
⅓ cup water
⅛ teaspoon freshly ground pepper
⅛ teaspoon ground allspice
2 teaspoons mild-flavored honey

Combine the mustard seeds, white wine or vermouth, vinegar, and 1 teaspoon of the tarragon in a bowl and let stand for at least 3 hours.

Pour the mixture into a blender jar or food processor (a blender does a more thorough job, if you have the patience to stop and start and stir the mixture) and add the remaining ingredients except the additional teaspoon of tarragon. Purée as finely as you can.

Scrape into the top part of a double boiler and stir over simmering water for about 10 minutes. A layer will stick to the bottom of the pan, but don't get alarmed—it won't burn as long as you are using a double boiler. Cool, add the remaining tarragon, and scrape into a jar. Refrigerate.

Tomato Catsup
Makes 1 quart

The kind of catsup most of us grew up eating contains significant amounts of both salt and sugar. But there's no reason why you can't make your own catsup, and you might like it even better than the commercial variety. This won't be quite as sweet and spicy as you may be accustomed to, but it is just as satisfying. Eaten with tofu, it will transport you back to your burger days.

Before preparing this recipe and the chili and chutneys that follow, you may want to consult a canning reference for instructions on canning. *Joy of Cooking*, the *USDA Canning Book*, *Putting Food By*, and *Better Than Store-Bought* all have sections that contain very detailed information about canning and preserving.

4 quarts ripe, fleshy tomatoes, preferably Italian plum variety
1 onion, minced
½ medium sweet red pepper, minced
2 cloves garlic, minced or put through a press
1 cup cider vinegar
2 teaspoons mustard seeds
2 teaspoons whole allspice berries
1 stick cinnamon, broken up
1 teaspoon whole black peppercorns
1 bay leaf
½ teaspoon whole cloves
½ ground coriander (cilantro)
⅛ teaspoon dried red pepper flakes
¼ cup mild-flavored honey or apple concentrate

Quarter the tomatoes and boil in a large saucepan for 30 minutes, stirring occasionally. Measure 2 quarts of the pulp into a large stainless steel or enameled pot. Add the onion, sweet red pepper, garlic, and vinegar and bring to a boil.

Tie the mustard seeds, allspice, cinnamon, peppercorns, bay leaf, cloves, coriander, and pepper flakes together in doubled cheesecloth. Add to the tomatoes, along with the honey or apple concentrate. Simmer uncovered for 1 hour over medium heat, stirring often.

Remove the cheesecloth bag and squeeze out all the moisture. Purée the tomato mixture in a blender, then press through a sieve or put through the fine blade of a food mill. Return to the pot and simmer over low heat until the mixture is thick enough to mound up slightly on a spoon. (It will thicken further upon cooling.)

Ladle into 2 clean, sterilized pint jars or 1 quarter jar, leaving ½ inch headspace. Wipe the rims and cover with canning jar lids.

Put the jars on a rack in a kettle half full of boiling water; add more boiling water to cover the lids by 2 inches. Bring to a hard boil, cover the pot, and boil for 15 minutes for pint jars, 20 minutes for quarts.

Remove from the boiling water and allow to cool. Let mellow in the jars for 2 to 4 weeks. Once opened, keep refrigerated. Store unopened jars in a cool, dry place.

Tomato Relish

Makes 1½ quarts

This is like the catsup above, but chunkier and more spicy. Relish and catsup can be used interchangeably.

    3 quarts ripe, meaty tomatoes, peeled (see Note)
    2 medium onions, finely minced
    2 red or green peppers, seeds removed, finely minced
    2 cups cider or distilled white vinegar
    ⅓ cup mild-flavored honey or apple concentrate
    1½ teaspoons mustard seeds
    1 teaspoon whole cloves
    2 teaspoons broken-up cinnamon stick
    1½ teaspoons whole allspice
    ¾ teaspoon black peppercorns
    1 clove garlic, peeled and left whole

Combine the tomatoes, onions, and peppers in a large stainless steel or enameled pot and bring to a simmer. Cook for about 30 minutes, until the onion is translucent. Add the vinegar and honey or apple concentrate and continue to cook over medium heat.

Place all the spices and the garlic together in a double thickness of cheesecloth and add to the pot. Continue to cook, uncovered, stirring from time to time and pressing the spice bag against the side of the pot to help extract flavors, for about 1½ hours. The sauce should reduce by almost half, and should have a chunky texture. It will tend to splatter, so don't lean over the pot.

Remove the spice bag, pressing against the side of the pot to extract the juices, and continue to cook the sauce, stirring, until quite thick. It should release no liquid when a spoonful is put on a plate.

Ladle into clean, sterilized pint jars, wipe the rim, and cap with canning lids. Place on a rack in a deep kettle full of boiling water and add more water to cover by 2 inches. Bring to a hard boil and cover the pot. Process for 15 minutes and remove from the boiling water. Allow to cool. Let mellow in the jars for 2 to 4 weeks before eating. Refrigerate once opened. Store unopened jars in a cool, dry place.

Note: To peel tomatoes, drop into boiling water for 20 seconds, drain, and run under cold water.

Tomato Chutney
Makes 1 quart

    1 pound apples, peeled, cored, and chopped
    2 pounds fresh ripe tomatoes, chopped
    2 ounces fresh ginger, finely minced or grated
    1 cup cider vinegar
    1 small onion, minced
    1 tablespoon raisins
    1 teaspoon ground cardamom
    ½ teaspoon powdered cloves
    2 tablespoons mild-flavored honey

Combine all the ingredients in a stainless steel or enameled saucepan and simmer 1 hour, uncovered. Ladle into hot, sterilized pint jars, wipe the rims, and seal with canning lids. Process in boiling water for 15 minutes. Cool. Refrigerate once opened. Store unopened jars in a cool, dark place:

Mixed Fruit Chutney
Makes 2 quarts

> 1 cup cider vingear
> ⅓ cup mild-flavored honey
> 1 clove garlic, minced or put through a press
> 1½ teaspoons freshly grated ginger root or ¾ teaspoon ground dried
> ¼ teaspoon freshly ground pepper
> ½ teaspoon ground cinnamon
> 1 tablespoon mustard seeds
> ½ teaspoon ground cloves
> ½ teaspoon ground coriander (cilantro)
> 2 medium tomatoes, peeled (see Note) and diced
> ½ onion, chopped fine
> 2 apples, peeled and diced
> 2 pears, peeled and diced
> ¼ cup raisins
> ¼ cup chopped figs

Combine all the ingredients in a large enameled or stainless steel saucepan and bring to a boil. Reduce heat, cover, and simmer for 2 hours, until you have a chutney with a thick consistency.

Transfer to hot, sterilized jars and process in a boiling water bath for 20 minutes. Cool and store in a cool, dry place. Once opened, keep refrigerated.

Note: To peel tomatoes, drop into boiling water for 20 seconds, drain, and run under cold water.

20. Miscellaneous Recipes

The recipes that follow don't really fit into a category, but most of them will come up in the menus from time to time.

Homemade Nonfat Yogurt
Makes 1 quart

Even the low-fat yogurts that are sold in supermarkets and health food stores contain a certain amount of high-fat milk solids. However, Colombo has begun marketing a completely nonfat yogurt that is available in some cities. The solution is to make your own. You only need to buy one cup of Dannon plain yogurt to use as the "starter." Once you make your own, you can use it to start the next batch.

There is nothing complicated about making yogurt at home. You do not need any fancy equipment or special yogurtmakers, and you don't need to scald milk. All you need is a blender, a big pot that is tall enough to contain the jars, and a low heat source. This can be a pilot light, a very low burner or a low burner covered with an asbestos pad or "flame tamer," an oven with a pilot light, a space heater, a cooler full of warm water, or even an electric blanket with a medium-low setting.

If the yogurt fails it is probably because your starter wasn't strong enough, or your waterbath was too hot or too cold. Don't let one failure deter you from trying again. Sometimes it takes a few tries to get the feel for it.

Because you're using nonfat dry milk for this yogurt, it contains very little fat—and you can make it at a fraction of the cost of the commercial product.

> 3½ cups lukewarm water (95°–110°F)
> 1 heaping cup spray-dried nonfat dry milk, or 1½ envelopes Sanalac commercial spray-dried milk
> 2–3 tablespoons *plain* yogurt (unflavored), such as Dannon

Place 2 cups of the lukewarm water in your blender jar along with the plain yogurt. Turn on the blender and pour in the spray-dried milk. Blend until the milk is dissolved, just about 10 to 15 seconds. Pour in the remaining warm water, and transfer the mixture into a quart jar or two pint jars and cover with a tight-fitting lid.

Place the jar in a pan of lukewarm water. The pan must be tall enough so that the water covers the entire jar. Cover and place in a warm spot where the temperature will remain constant, such as over a pilot light, on a heater, or in a cooler full of warm water. You could also wrap the jar in an electric blanket set medium-low. If the weather is warm, leave for about 4 hours. In cold weather it will take at least 6 hours. Check from time to time to make sure the water doesn't become too hot, or cool off, and adjust the temperature as necessary by adding hot or cold water. Refrigerate when thick. Always save a couple of tablespoons to start the next batch.

Nutty Tofu Cheese Substitute

Makes 1½ cups

This can be substituted for cheese in casseroles. It bakes to a golden brown. Instead of bubbling like cheese, it firms up. It will keep for about 5 days in the refrigerator, but it does not freeze well, since it contains tofu.

> ½ pound (2 cakes) tofu
> ½ cup Homemade Nonfat Yogurt (page 217)
> 2 tablespoons sesame tahini
> 1–2 tablespoons lemon juice, to taste
> freshly grated nutmeg to taste
> 1–2 teaspoons grated fresh ginger (optional)

Blend all the ingredients together in a food processor or blender until completely smooth. Transfer to a covered container and chill.

Sprouts

Growing sprouts is like growing a garden in your kitchen. The crop you will harvest, in 3 days, is one of nature's most concentrated, low-calorie sources of protein and other nutrients. The nutrients contained in sprouts correspond to those contained in unsprouted beans or seeds; but the proteins occur in a simpler form and are more readily available. (They can be metabolized more quickly.) In addition to the proteins and carbohydrates that sprouts will provide you, you will obtain from them many vitamins and minerals—especially A, B, C, and E—because each sprout is both a small leafy vegetable and a bean or seed. Alfalfa seeds, mung beans, lentils, black beans, azuki beans, wheat berries, whole triticale, whole rye, and sunflower seeds all make good sprouts. Each kind tastes unique.

There is no trick to making sprouts at home, and you need no fancy equipment. A wide, flat baking dish covered with a towel will work very well.

FIRST NIGHT, OR DAY
¼ cup seeds or beans, such as alfalfa, mung, lentil (these are the easiest)
1 cup water
a jar or measuring cup

Soak the seeds or beans in the water, in jar or measuring cup, overnight, or for at least 10 hours.

DAY 2
a strainer
a wide, flat dish, nonmetallic and not low-fire glazed, or a wide-mouth jar with a flat side
paper towels
a dish towel
cheesecloth for jar

Drain the seeds or beans in strainer, rinse with cold water, and drain again. Place in the wide, flat dish in a single layer, making sure they are not sitting in water. Cover with a damp layer of paper towels, and cover the dish with a towel.

If you are using a jar, place the seeds or beans in the jar and cover the mouth with a layer of cheesecloth attached with a rubber band or with a sprouting lid, easily available in health food stores. Shake the jar so that the seeds or beans adhere to the sides and don't all pile up on top of each other. Wrap the jar in a towel and lay it on its side.

Rinse the seeds or beans throughly twice a day with cool water. You are actually watering the seeds so that they'll grow, so water and drain thoroughly or the seeds will either dry out or rot. If you are using a dish, cover again with paper toweling and a dish towel.

DAYS 3–5

Continue rinsing twice a day. Wheat berries and other grains will be ready to refrigerate by the third day. Most of the others will be ready by the fourth. The sprouts should be 2 or 3 times the length of the seed (longer for many), and roots should not have begun to develop.

When the sprouts are ready, place in the sun for a couple of hours to bring out the chlorophyll. Then refrigerate in plastic bags for up to a week.

Fruit and Sprout Smoothie
Makes 1 drink

> Salads aren't the only places for sprouts. You can blend a large quantity with fruit juice and mint for a terrific breakfast, lunch, or snack.

1 cup orange or apple juice
½ cup alfalfa sprouts
2 tablespoons fresh mint
½ banana
2 ice cubes

Blend all the ingredients together in the blender until smooth.

Roasted Soybeans
Makes 1 cup

These are nothing like the salty and oily commercial variety. The cruchiness and deep-roasted flavor add interest to salads and casseroles. They also make a good snack.

Roasted soybeans can also be cracked in a blender and sprinkled onto casseroles or vegetable dishes, or added to salads or sandwiches. They have an almost baconlike flavor. If you ate the Roasted Soybean, Sprouts, and Tomato Sandwich (page 285) blindfolded, you might think you were eating a bacon, lettuce, and tomato sandwich.

   1 cup dried soybeans, washed, picked over, and soaked
   3 cups water

Combine the soybeans and water in a large saucepan (at least twice their volume, as they expand substantially) and bring to a boil. Cover, reduce heat, and simmer 1 hour. Drain.

Preheat the oven to 325 degrees.

Spread the beans on a baking sheet or in a baking pan and place in the preheated oven. Bake for 1 to 1½ hours, turning every 15 minutes and checking carefully when the soybeans begin to smell toasty. To see if they are done, remove one from the pan, let it cool, and bite through. If it isn't crunchy all the way through, bake about 10 to 15 minutes longer. Be careful as soon as soybeans begin to smell toasty, because they burn quickly once they are done. Remove from the oven when ready and allow to cool. Store in a tightly sealed jar. They will keep this way for months in a cool, dry place.

Meatless Chili—Terlingua Style
Serves 4 to 6

This recipe was devised by Mr. Tom Griffin, 1977 Terlingua Chili Festival King and participant in our study.

Serve this chili over cooked pinto or kidney beans, if desired. It may also be used for filling in tacos or enchiladas. Many people like chili with a small amount of grated low-fat cheese or toasted tortilla chips.

two 8-ounce cans unsalted tomato sauce, if available
4 cups water
1 medium onion, chopped
4–5 cloves garlic, minced
2 ounces chili powder
3–5 dashes of cayenne pepper, or to taste
¼ teaspoon ground oregano
dash of paprika
2 cups textured vegetable protein (available in health food
   stores)
¼ teaspoon ground cumin
masa (corn flour) or corn meal as needed.

Place the tomato sauce and 4 cups of water in a deep 6- to 8-quart pot. Add onion and garlic. Bring to a boil. Reduce heat and simmer for 30 minutes. Add chili powder, cayenne, oregano, and paprika, stirring well. Add textured vegetable protein, stir well, and simmer for 30 minutes, stirring occasionally. Add water as needed. Stir in cumin, add water if needed for desired consistency, and cook for 5 more minutes. If additional thickness is desired, stir 1 tablespoon of masa (corn flour) into the chili. Corn meal may be substituted for masa. Cook 8 to 10 minutes after adding the masa.

Homemade Granola

Makes 2½ quarts

For most of us, "breakfast" and "cereal" are two words that belong together. Unfortunately, most of the commercially available cereals are loaded with salt, sugar, and oil. Shredded Wheat by Nabisco and Puffed Wheat and Puffed Rice by Quaker are commercial cereals that do not contain added salt or sugar. A few others can be found in health food stores, including some marketed by the Health Valley Company. When you shop, be sure to read the labels—even "natural" cereals are often loaded with salt, sugar, and oil.

The granola recipe below has no added salt and only a small amount of honey and oil. The vanilla, spices, and raisins give it a sweet flavor. If you are unable to find flaked wheat, rye, or triticale, then just add more oats.

As for what to put on the granola, a little nonfat yogurt and some fresh fruit are delicious. The Sweet Yogurt Cereal Topping on page 202 also works well; so does apple juice diluted with an equal amount of water.

3 cups rolled oats
1½ cups flaked wheat
1½ cups flaked rye or flaked triticale
3 cups untoasted wheat germ
1 teaspoon powdered cinnamon
1 teaspoon nutmeg
½ cup soy flour
3 tablespoons sesame seeds
3 tablespoons sunflower seeds
1 tablespoon vanilla extract
¼ cup safflower oil
¼ cup mild-flavored honey or malt syrup
½ cup raisins

Preheat oven to 250 degrees.

Mix together all the dry ingredients, except the raisins, with the vanilla.

Stir together the safflower oil and the honey or syrup, then add the grains. Toss thoroughly, mixing until the oil and honey are evenly distributed and there are no lumps.

Place in a large baking pan and bake in the low oven for 2 hours, stirring to redistribute the grains every 20 minutes. Add the raisins during the last 20 minutes. Cool in the pan and refrigerate in a tightly sealed jar. (This granola keeps best in the refrigerator.)

21. Three Weeks of Menus

Below are three weeks of menus based on the meals that were served during our research study.

If possible, your big meal should be the midday one, but this is unrealistic for many of us. So, you may want to switch the order of lunches and dinners, or to streamline meals wherever you desire.

Some of the lunches in these menus are quick and simple. Others may be longer or demand more cooking time than you are accustomed to. These menus are merely *suggestions*. You can elaborate on them or simplify. You may be more comfortable with foods from Goups 1 and 2 with which you are more familiar. For easier meals, eat steamed vegetables with one of the sauces (Chapter 18), grains (Chapter 15), salads, and legumes (Chapter 15).

Certain foods on the menus, like the Fresh Orange Juice on Day 1 and Corn on the Cob on Day 3, are self-explanatory and therefore no recipe has been provided.

If a recipe has already been presented in Chapters 15–20, it is not repeated in the menus. Once a recipe is given under one day's menu, it is not repeated when suggested for a later date. In both these instances, cross-references are provided.

All of these menus have been verified for nutritional adequacy.

DAY 1

BREAKFAST
> *Oatmeal with Apples, Spices, and Raisins*
> *Fresh Orange Juice*

LUNCH
> *Baked Potatoes with Yogurt*
> *Spinach Salad*
> *Watermelon with Lime Juice*

DINNER
> *Spaghetti with Tomato-Vegetable Sauce*
> *Tossed Green Salad*
> *Whole Wheat Sage and Onion Bread (page 180)*
> *Bananas Poached in Apple Juice*

RECIPES

Oatmeal with Apples, Spices and Raisins
Serves 4

> 2 cups water
> 1 cup oatmeal
> 3 tablespoons raisins
> ½–1 teaspoon ground cinnamon
> ½ teaspoon nutmeg (freshly grated if possible)
> 1 apple, grated and tossed with the juice of ½ lemon
> 1 tablespoon Homemade Nonfat Yogurt (page 217) per serving
> additional cinnamon (optional)

Place the water in a saucepan and bring to a rolling boil. Slowly pour in the oatmeal, stirring all the while with a wooden spoon. Add the raisins, cinnamon, and nutmeg, bring to a second boil, and reduce the heat. Cover and simmer 15 to 20 minutes, or until the liquid is absorbed. Top each serving with grated apple, a dollop of yogurt, and, if you desire, additional ground cinnamon.

Baked Potatoes with Yogurt
Serves 4

Baked potatoes do not have to be drowning in butter to be delicious—there are plenty of other foods with which to moisten them. Yogurt is just one possibility.

Here is a simple version of the dish.

    4 baking potatoes
    1 cup Homemade Nonfat Yogurt (page 217)
    freshly ground pepper to taste

OPTIONAL

    1 teaspoon ground cumin
    1 teaspoon curry powder
    1 teaspoon caraway seeds
    1 tablespoon chopped fresh herbs, such as parsley, basil,
        dill, thyme, marjoram
    lemon juice to taste

Preheat oven to 425 degrees. Puncture the potato skins with a fork and bake 40 minutes to an hour, until tender.

Slit the potatoes open and top with yogurt, either plain or flavored with one of the suggestions above. Add plenty of freshly ground black pepper.

Note: You can also season your yogurt with garlic, other spices or herbs, or even a cup of puréed, steamed vegetable, like cauliflower, broccoli, carrots, or peas. If you don't like the taste of yogurt, don't despair. Try unsalted tomato juice or tomato sauce. If you have a soup on hand, blend up some of it and use as a "gravy." Or you may wish to try one of the sauces on pages 200–07 that appeals to you. Salsa Fresca and Simple Tomato Sauce are particularly good.

Spinach Salad

Serves 6

> ½ pound fresh spinach, washed carefully, stems removed, and dried
> 4 fresh mushrooms, wiped clean and sliced
> 4 green onions, both white and green parts, sliced
> 1 cup alfalfa sprouts
> 2 tablespoons sunflower seeds

Toss all ingredients. For salad dressing, try the Yogurt Vinaigrette (page 195).

Spaghetti with Tomato-Vegetable Sauce

Serves 6

> 2 teaspoons safflower oil
> 1 onion, chopped
> 2–4 cloves garlic, to taste, minced or put through a press
> 1 medium-sized carrot, grated
> 1 cup sliced fresh mushrooms
> ¼ teaspoon dried thyme
> 2 pounds fresh ripe tomatoes, chopped
> 6 ounces unsalted tomato paste
> 1 medium zucchini, sliced ¼ inch thick
> 1 tablespoon chopped fresh basil or parsley
> 1 teaspoon dried basil
> pinch of cinnamon
> freshly ground pepper
> pinch of cayenne pepper (optional)
> 1 pound whole grain spaghetti
> additional fresh herbs (up to 3 tablespoons), such as parsley or basil, for garnish

In a large, heavy-bottomed saucepan or Dutch oven (preferably nonstick), heat the safflower oil and sauté the onion with half the garlic until the onion is just tender (about 3 minutes). Add the carrot and mushrooms and sauté another few minutes, until the mushrooms begin to soften. Add the thyme and continue to sauté (for a minute or so), stirring. Add the tomatoes and tomato paste. Turn heat to medium and bring to a simmer. Simmer, stirring from time to time, for 30 minutes. Add the zucchini and remaining garlic, the herbs, and cinnamon, and continue to simmer for 20 to 30 minutes. Add freshly ground pepper to taste, and more herbs if you wish. This sauce will freeze well and will keep several days in the refrigerator in a covered container.

Fill a large pot with at least 6 quarts of water and bring to a boil. Add the spaghetti and give it a stir. Cook al dente—that is, until spaghetti is soft but still firm to the bite. (With whole grain noodles this takes anywhere from 4 to 10 minutes.) After 4 minutes, begin testing the noodles by removing one and biting into it. It should be neither starchy nor mushy.

Remove the spaghetti from the water with a slotted spoon or deep-fry skimmer (or you can drain the spaghetti in a colander, but it will not remain as hot) and place in a warm serving dish. Top with the sauce, garnish with fresh herbs if you wish, and serve at once.

Tossed Green Salad

Serves 4 to 6

> ¾ pound lettuce, Boston, leaf, romaine, or red tip or a combination
> ½ cucumber, sliced thin
> 4 radishes, sliced thin
> 4 mushrooms, sliced thin
> 3 green onions, both white and green parts, sliced
> 1–2 tablespoons fresh herbs, if available (such as basil, thyme, dill, parsley, marjoram, fennel)
> ½–1 cup alfalfa, mung bean, or lentil sprouts
> Low-Fat Vinaigrette of your choice (pages 195–97)

OPTIONAL

> sliced tomatoes or cherry tomatoes
> cooked garbanzos or other beans
> cubed tofu
> sliced green pepper
> leftover cooked grains, such as rice, bulgur, wheat berries, rye, couscous
> leftover or freshly steamed vegetables, such as broccoli, cauliflower, zucchini, green beans, corn, beets
> Whole Grain Croutons (page 184)

Toss together all the ingredients except the dressing, adding any of the optional ingredients you like. Toss with the dressing just before serving.

Bananas Poached in Apple Juice
Serves 4 to 6

>2 cups apple juice
>juice of ½ lemon
>¼ cup raisins
>1 tablespoon vanilla extract
>3-inch stick of cinnamon
>3 ripe but firm bananas
>freshly grated nutmeg to taste
>½ cup Homemade Nonfat Yogurt (page 217)

Combine the apple juice, lemon juice, raisins, vanilla, and cinnamon in a 4- or 5-quart saucepan and bring to a simmer. Simmer 5 minutes. Peel the bananas and slice into the mixture. Simmer another 10 minutes. Sprinkle on fresh nutmeg and serve, garnishing each serving with a dollop of yogurt. The bananas can be served hot, warm, or at room temperature. Serve the leftovers for breakfast, on hot cereal, or with additional yogurt.

DAY 2

BREAKFAST
> *Corn Meal Muffins*
> *Half Grapefruit*

LUNCH
> *Steamed Spinach*
> *Brown Rice (page 169)*
> *Green Bean Salad*
> *Sliced Fresh Strawberries*

DINNER
> *Lettuce and Citrus Salad*
> *Deep-Dish Vegetable Pie*
> *Pineapple with Mint*

RECIPES

Corn Meal Muffins
Makes 12 to 14 muffins

> 4 teaspoons active dry yeast
> ½ cup lukewarm water
> 2 tablespoons plus ½ teaspoon mild-flavored honey
> ¾ cup stone-ground corn meal
> 1 cup whole wheat flour
> ½ cup Homemade Nonfat Yogurt (page 217)
> 2 tablespoons safflower oil, plus additional for muffin tins

Dissolve the yeast in the warm water in a small bowl, along with ½ teaspoon honey. Let sit 10 minutes.

Combine the corn meal and whole wheat flour and sift into a mixing bowl.

In another bowl mix together the yogurt, 2 tablespoons honey, and 2 tablespoons safflower oil. When the yeast has begun to foam, stir it into the yogurt mixture.

Stir the liquid mixture into the flours with just four or five stirs. The batter should be lumpy.

Fill lightly oiled muffin tins two-thirds full. Set in a draft-free area and let rise 30 minutes. Meanwhile preheat the oven to 375 degrees.

Bake the muffins in the preheated oven for 25 minutes. Let cool in the tins for 10 minutes, then remove, running a knife around the edges of the muffins if they stick to the pan, and cool on racks, or serve hot, with Apple Spice Tofu Morning Spread (page 192).

Steamed Squash
Serves 4

> 1½ pounds summer squash—yellow squash or zucchini or a combination
> fresh chopped herbs, such as parsley, basil, thyme, rosemary, dill, or marjoram (up to 1 tablespoon) (optional)
> ½ teaspoon dried herbs, such as tarragon, thyme, dill, or rosemary (optional)
> freshly ground pepper to taste
> lemon wedges

Steam the squash for 10 minutes in a covered saucepan. Place in a serving dish and toss with, if you wish, fresh or dried herbs and with plenty of freshly ground pepper. Serve with lemon wedges so that each person can season to taste with lemon juice.

Green Bean Salad
Serves 4 to 6

> 1 pound green breans, trimmed and cut in half if very long
> 3 tablespoons chopped fresh parsley
> 3–4 mushrooms, wiped clean and sliced
> 2 tablespoons chopped fresh chives or green onion tops
> Low-Fat Vinaigrette (page 195) or choose a variation, such as Tomato Vinaigrette (page 196)

Steam the beans in a covered saucepan for 5 to 10 minutes, until crisp-tender and bright green. Softness will depend on your taste. Refresh under cold water. Toss with the parsley, mushrooms, chopped chives or green onion tops, and the vinaigrette of your choice. Serve at once, or chill and serve.

231

Sliced Fresh Strawberries

Serves 4

>1 pint fresh strawberries, washed, hulled, and sliced
>1 tablespoon black cherry concentrate (optional)
>½ cup Homemade Nonfat Yogurt (page 217) (optional)
>1 tablespoon fresh mint leaves

Toss sliced strawberries with optional black cherry concentrate. Arrange in bowls and garnish each serving with a dollop of yogurt and a few leaves of fresh mint.

Lettuce and Citrus Salad

Serves 6

>½ head romaine lettuce
>¼ cup sliced green onions
>Low-Fat Vinaigrette or Yogurt Vinaigrette (page 195)
>2 oranges, peeled and cut in sections
>1 tablespoon pecans

Toss the lettuce and green onions with all but 2 tablespoons of the vinaigrette. Place in a salad bowl. Toss the oranges and pecans with the remaining dressing and scatter over the lettuce leaves.

Deep-Dish Vegetable Pie

Serves 6 to 8

FOR THE CRUST
>1 tablespoon active dry yeast
>¼ cup lukewarm water
>½ teaspoon mild-flavored honey
>1 tablespoon safflower oil, plus additional
>3½–4 cups whole wheat flour, as needed
>corn meal

FOR THE SAUCE
>2 cups whole mushrooms
>1½ cups water
>½ cup dry white wine
>4 whole cloves garlic
>¼–½ teaspoon dried thyme, to taste
>freshly ground pepper to taste
>pinch of cayenne pepper

FOR THE FILLING

2 teaspoons safflower oil
1 onion, thinly sliced
2 cloves garlic, minced or put through a press
2 cups sliced mushrooms
¼ cup dry white wine
¼ teaspoon dried thyme
freshly ground pepper to taste
1 cup broccoli florets
1 small zucchini, sliced ¼ inch thick
1 cup cauliflowerets
1 cup cooked soy flakes (½ cup raw; page 174)
3 tablespoons chopped fresh parsley
½–1 teaspoon dried oregano (or fresh, if available) to taste

Make the crust: Dissolve the yeast in the water with the honey in a large bowl. Let it sit for a while, then stir in 1 tablespoon safflower oil and 2 cups of the whole wheat flour, a cup at a time. Add another half cup of flour and fold it in. At this point the dough should be a rather sticky mass that can be turned out of the bowl. Place a cup of flour on your kneading surface and turn out the dough. Scrape whatever remains in the bowl onto the dough. Flour your hands and begin to knead by folding the dough in half toward you and leaning into the dough. Turn the dough a quarter turn, fold in half toward you, and lean into it. Turn, fold, lean. Continue kneading in this fashion, adding flour when the dough begins to stick to the kneading surface, until the dough is stiff and elastic—about 10 minutes. Oil the bowl lightly and place the dough in it, rounded surface down. Then turn the dough over so that the now oiled rounded surface is up. Cover with plastic or a moist towel and place in a warm place to rise for 1 to 1½ hours, until doubled in volume.

Punch down the dough by sticking your fist in the center a few times and turn out onto a lightly floured surface. Knead a few times and cut into two equal pieces, so that one piece is twice the size of the other.

Form the smaller piece into a ball, wrap in plastic, and refrigerate. Roll out the larger piece with a heavy rolling pin to ¼-inch thickness. Lightly oil a 3-quart baking dish and sprinkle with corn meal. Line it with the crust, and pinch a scalloped edge around the rim. Refrigerate while you prepare the filling. The dough can also be frozen at this point.

Begin the sauce: Combine the 2 cups whole mushrooms with the water, wine, and 4 whole cloves garlic in a saucepan. Simmer, covered, for 30 minutes, while you prepare the rest of the vegetables.

Prepare the filling: Heat the 2 teaspoons safflower oil in a heavy-bottomed skillet and sauté the onion with the garlic until the onion begins to soften. Add the sliced mushrooms and sauté 3 minutes. Add the ¼ cup white wine and the thyme and continue to sauté for 5 minutes, until the mushrooms are tender. Grind in some black pepper and remove from the heat.

Steam the broccoli, sliced zucchini, and cauliflower together for 5 minutes. Remove from the heat and toss with the sautéed mushrooms and onions. Stir in the soy flakes, parsley, and oregano.

Finish the sauce: Purée the simmered mushrooms and whole garlic in their liquid and add thyme, freshly ground pepper, and cayenne.

Preheat the oven to 400 degress. Prebake the crust for 5 minutes. Remove from the heat and turn the oven down to 350 degrees.

Fill the crust with the vegetable and soy flake combination. Pour in the sauce and distribute the vegetables evenly.

For a lattice, roll out the remaining piece of dough as thin as possible and cut in 1-inch strips. Weave them over the top of the dough and pinch over the edge.

Bake in preheated oven for 30 to 40 minutes, or until the crust is brown and the vegetables bubbling.

Pineapple with Mint
Serves 4

> ½ large or 1 small ripe pineapple
> 3 tablespoons chopped fresh mint

Here is a quick way to peel and chunk a whole pineapple. First cut the leaf end off the pineapple with a sharp stainless steel knife (carbon will discolor and give the fruit a metallic taste). Then cut the pineapple into quarters and run your knife down each quarter, just inside the skin so that the skin comes off in one neat piece. Cut away the core, and slice crosswise. Toss with the mint and serve, or chill and serve.

DAY 3

BREAKFAST

> *Banana-Yogurt Smoothie*
> *Toasted Herbed Triticale Bread (page 179) with Unsweetened Fruit Spread (either Apricot Preserves [page 193], Plum Sauce [page 208], or a commercial brand)*

LUNCH

> *Okra with Tomatoes*
> *Corn on the Cob*
> *Herbed Triticale Bread (page 179) with Mushroom Spread (page 188) or White Bean Spread (page 186)*
> *Tossed Green Salad (page 228)*
> *Sliced Apples with Lemon Juice*

DINNER

> *Middle Eastern Salad*
> *Eggplant and Rice Casserole*
> *Cantaloupe and Honeydew Slices*

RECIPES

Banana-Yogurt Smoothie

Makes 1 drink

> ½ cup Homemade Nonfat Yogurt (page 217)
> 1 small or ½ large banana
> ½ cup apple juice
> 2 ice cubes

Place all the ingredients in a blender and blend until smooth.

Okra with Tomatoes
Serves 4 to 6

>2 teaspoons safflower oil
>1 onion, chopped
>2 cloves garlic, minced or put through a press
>1½ pounds okra
>2 tablespoons vinegar
>1 pound tomatoes
>½ teaspoon dried basil or oregano

Heat the oil in a large nonstick or heavy-bottomed skillet and sauté the onion with the garlic until the onion begins to soften. Add the okra and the vinegar and sauté, stirring, for 5 minutes. Add the tomatoes and basil or oregano and continue to sauté, stirring from time to time, for another 10 to 15 minutes. Serve.

Sliced Apples with Lemon Juice
Serves 6

>3 apples
>juice of 1 lemon

Core and slice the apples and toss with the lemon juice. Refrigerate until ready to serve.

Middle Eastern Salad
Serves 6

>1 cucumber, peeled and chopped
>3 tomatoes, chopped
>4 green onions, both white and green parts, chopped
>½ cup chopped fresh mint
>½ cup chopped fresh parsley
>¾ cup mung bean sprouts
>½ cup lemon juice
>3 tablespoons cider or wine vinegar
>2 cloves garlic, minced or put through a press
>¾ cup Homemade Nonfat Yogurt (page 217)
>1 cup Whole Grain Croutons (page 184)

Toss together the cucumbers, tomatoes, green onions, mint, parsley, and bean sprouts in a salad bowl.

Mix together the lemon juice, vinegar, garlic, and yogurt and toss with the vegetables. Add the croutons, toss again, and serve, or refrigerate for an hour or two before adding the croutons and toss again with the croutons just before serving.

Eggplant and Rice Casserole
Serves 6 to 8

    3 cups cooked brown rice (page 169)
    ½ cup raw soy grits (page 169), cooked with the brown
      rice
    2 medium eggplants
    1 tablespoon safflower oil, plus additional for baking dishes
    1 medium to large onion, chopped
    1–2 cloves garlic, minced or put through a press
    1 cup sliced mushrooms
    1 green pepper, sliced
    ¼ cup dry white wine
    1 zucchini, sliced
    3 tomatoes, sliced
    ½ teaspoon allspice (more to taste)
    freshly ground pepper to taste
    ½ cup whole wheat bread crumbs
    ¼ cup chopped fresh parsley

Begin by cooking the rice and soy grits.

Preheat the oven to 450 degrees.

Cut the eggplant in half lengthwise, then score each half with a sharp knife down to the skin but not through it. Brush a baking sheet with safflower oil and lay the eggplants on it cut side down. Bake in the preheated oven for 15 to 20 minutes, while you prepare the other vegetables. Remove from the oven and allow to cool. When cool enough to handle, scoop out of the shells and dice. Set aside.

Reduce the oven temperature to 350 degrees.

Heat 1 tablespoon safflower oil in a nonstick or heavy-bottomed skillet and sauté the onion, garlic, mushrooms, and green pepper until the onion is tender. Add the eggplant and sauté, stirring, for

2 to 3 minutes, then add the wine, zucchini, and tomatoes. Cook over medium heat for 15 minutes, stirring occasionally. Add the allspice and freshly ground pepper and cook another 5 minutes.

Brush a 3- or 4-quart casserole or baking dish lightly with safflower oil and spread the rice and soy grits over the bottom. Cover the grains with the eggplant combination. Sprinkle the bread crumbs over the eggplant.

Bake 30 minutes in the preheated oven, until the bread crumbs brown and the casserole is bubbly. Remove, sprinkle on the parsley, and serve.

Cantaloupe and Honeydew Slices
Serves 6

½ ripe cantaloupe, thinly sliced
½ ripe honeydew, thinly sliced
juice of 1 lime
1 tablespoon minced fresh mint

Place melon slices on a platter, squeeze on lime juice, and sprinkle with mint.

DAY 4

BREAKFAST
> *Cream of Wheat with Raisins and Cinnamon*
> *Fresh Grapefruit Juice*

LUNCH
> *Sprouts, Tomato, and White Bean Spread Sandwich*
> *Steamed Broccoli*
> *Fruit Salad*

DINNER
> *Red Cabbage Salad with Poppy Seed Dressing*
> *Black-eyed Peas*
> *Yeasted Corn Bread (page 184)*
> *Frozen Banana Ice*

RECIPES

Cream of Wheat with Raisins and Cinnamon
Serves 4

> 3 cups water
> 1 cup Cream of Wheat
> 1 teaspoon cinnamon
> ¼ cup raisins
> 1 cup Sweet Yogurt Cereal Topping (page 202)

Bring the water to a boil in a saucepan. Slowly pour in the Cream of Wheat in a very slow stream, stirring all the time with a wooden spoon. Add the cinnamon and raisins, bring to a second boil, reduce heat, and cover. Cook 15 minutes, or until the liquid is absorbed. Top each serving with not more than ¼ cup topping.

Sprouts, Tomato, and White Bean Spread Sandwich

Makes 1 sandwich

1 slice Herbed Triticale Bread (page 179) or Whole Wheat Sage and Onion Bread (page 180)
1 tablespoon White Bean Spread (page 186)
2 slices ripe tomato
2 tablespoons alfalfa sprouts
2 teaspoons Roasted Soybeans (page 221), cracked in a blender
1 teaspoon vinegar

Spread each slice of bread with the white bean spread, then top with slices of ripe tomato, alfalfa sprouts, cracked roasted soybeans, and vinegar.

Steamed Broccoli

Serves 4

2 cups broccoli pieces, steamed until crisp-tender
lemon juice to taste

Steam the broccoli 10 minutes, toss with the lemon juice, and serve.

Fruit Salad

Serves 4

1 peach, sliced
1 plum, sliced
1 apple, sliced
1 banana, sliced
¼ teaspoon ground cardamom
juice of 1 lime

Toss together the fruit, cardamom, and lime juice. Serve at room temperature or chilled.

Red Cabbage Salad with Poppy Seed Dressing

Serves 4 to 6

⅓ cup lemon juice
2 tablespoons apple juice
2 tablespoons cider vinegar
2 tablespoons poppy seeds
¾ cup Homemade Nonfat Yogurt (page 217)
4 cups shredded red cabbage
leaf lettuce for the bowl

Combine the lemon juice, apple juice, cider vinegar, and poppy seeds and stir in the yogurt. Toss with the shredded red cabbage. Line a salad bowl with the lettuce leaves and fill with the cabbage. Serve chilled or at room temperature.

Black-eyed Peas

Serves 6 to 8

Black-eyed peas have a distinctive, soothing flavor. They require no soaking and take comparatively little time to cook.

2 teaspoons safflower oil
1 medium or large onion, chopped
3 cloves garlic, minced or put through a press
1 pound black-eyed peas, washed and picked over
6 cups water
1 bay leaf
1 pound tomatoes, chopped
1 teaspoon oregano or 1 tablespoon chopped fresh herbs
    such as basil, parsley, or marjoram (optional)
freshly ground pepper

Heat the oil in a large, heavy-bottomed saucepan and sauté the onion with 1 clove of garlic until the onion is tender. Add the black-eyed peas, the water, and the bay leaf and bring to a boil. Cover, reduce heat, and simmer 30 minutes. Add the tomatoes, herbs, and remaining garlic and continue to simmer another 30 minutes, or until the peas are tender. Add freshly ground pepper to taste, and serve with hot corn bread. Black-eyed peas also go well with corn on the cob.

Frozen Banana Ice
Serves 4 to 6

> 4 bananas, peeled and frozen
> 1 cup Homemade Nonfat Yogurt (page 217)
> 2 teaspoons vanilla extract
> freshly grated nutmeg to taste

Peel and freeze the bananas. (They will take 24 hours to freeze solid.)

Place the frozen bananas, yogurt, and vanilla in the bowl of a food processor and pulse about 20 times until the bananas are broken up into fairly uniform pieces. Continue to process until you have a smooth ice, about 30 seconds to a minute. Season to taste with freshly grated nutmeg.

Serve at once, or chill in the freezer for up to an hour—any longer and the mixture will become frozen solid. If it does solidify, remove from the freezer and place in the refrigerator for 1 hour before serving.

DAY 5

BREAKFAST

Homemade Granola (page 222) with Sweet Yogurt Cereal Topping (page 202)

LUNCH

Steamed Peas and Cauliflower
Potato-Caraway Salad
Herbed Triticale Bread (page 217) or Whole Wheat Sage and Onion Bread (page 218)
Fresh Pears, Sliced or Whole

DINNER

Saffron Millet
Vegetable Shish Kebab
Shredded Carrot Salad with Poppy Seed Dressing
Tofu Banana Cream Pie

RECIPES

Steamed Peas and Cauliflower

Serves 4

Not only do these two vegetables taste good together, they also look beautiful. If you can't find fresh peas, use frozen, but choose an unsalted, unbuttered brand.

    1 small head cauliflower, broken into pieces
    1 cup shelled peas (1 pound unshelled) or 1 cup frozen,
        thawed
    lemon juice (optional)
    chopped fresh herbs (optional)

Steam the cauliflower for 10 minutes. Add the peas and steam another 5 to 10 minutes, to taste. Toss with lemon juice and fresh herbs if desired.

Potato-Caraway Salad
Serves 6

> 1½ pounds new or russet potatoes
> ¼ cup dry white wine
> 1 Bermuda onion, poached if desired (see Note) and sliced thin
> 2 teaspoons caraway seeds
> 2 tablespoons chopped fresh parsley
> juice of 1 lemon
> ¼ cup cider vinegar
> ½ teaspoon ground mustard or 1 teaspoon Homemade Mustard Without Salt (page 211)
> 1 clove garlic, minced or put through a press
> 2 tablespoons safflower oil
> ½ cup water

Cut the potatoes in half and steam until just tender (about 20 minutes). Refresh under cold water and slice. Toss immediately with the white wine, sliced onion, caraway seeds, and parsley.

Mix together the lemon juice, vinegar, mustard, and garlic. Whisk in the safflower oil, then the water. Toss with the potatoes and serve chilled or warm.

Note: Poaching onions renders them milder in flavor. To poach, place onion in a pot of water, bring to a boil, and boil 3 minutes. Drain and refresh under cold water.

Saffron Millet
Serves 4

This doesn't taste much different from plain millet (see cooking instructions, page 169), but it has a beautiful saffron hue. Currants add variety.

> 1 teaspoon safflower oil
> 1 cup millet
> 2 cups simmering water
> ½ teaspoon Spanish saffron
> ¼ cup currants (optional)

Heat the oil in a heavy-bottomed saucepan and sauté the millet for about 3 minutes (until it begins to smell toasty). Pour in the simmering water, stirring, and add the saffron. If you like currants, add these now. Cover, reduce heat, and simmer 30 minutes. Uncover and continue to simmer 5 to 10 more minutes until all the liquid has evaporated.

Vegetable Shish Kebab
Serves 4

These kebabs make attractive food. The marinade is pungent with curry and onion. Serve the kebabs over hot, cooked millet or saffron millet.

FOR THE MARINADE
3 cups Homemade Nonfat Yogurt (page 217)
1½ cups water
1 onion, grated
4 cloves garlic, minced or put through a press
2 tablespoons grated fresh ginger
2 tablespoon curry powder (more to taste)
freshly ground pepper to taste
2 teaspoons ground cumin
juice of 1 lemon

FOR THE VEGETABLES
½ pint cherry tomatoes
2 green peppers, seeded and quartered or cut in lengths
2 onions, cut in eighths or quartered
½ pound firm, fresh mushrooms, stems removed
1 medium zucchini, sliced ½ inch thick
2 medium potatoes, unpeeled, cut in chunks, and steamed
    10 minutes, or until crisp-tender
1 yellow squash, sliced ½ inch thick

Combine all the ingredients for the marinade in a large bowl. Prepare the vegetables and toss with the marinade. Refrigerate and marinate for several hours, tossing at intervals to distribute the marinade evenly.

Prepare a fire in your grill/barbecue pit, or preheat the oven to 400 degrees, or light the broiler.

Place the marinated vegetables on skewers, alternating them to make a colorful arrangement. Roast the kebabs over the open fire, in the hot oven, or under the broiler, basting often with the leftover marinade. This should take 20 to 30 minutes. Make sure to turn the skewers from time to time to ensure even cooking.

Shredded Carrot Salad with Poppy Seed Dressing
Serves 4 to 6

    juice of ½ lemon
    2 tablespoons mild-flavored honey
    2 tablespoons cider vinegar
    2 tablespoons poppy seeds
    ½ cup Homemade Nonfat Yogurt (page 217)
    1 pound carrots, scrubbed and grated
    leaf lettuce for the bowl
    2 tablespoons safflower seeds

Mix together the lemon juice, honey, vinegar, poppy seeds, and yogurt. Toss with the grated carrots. Line a salad bowl with the lettuce leaves and fill with the carrots. Sprinkle on the sunflower seeds and serve, or chill and serve.

Tofu Banana Cream Pie
Serves 8 to 10

People often can't believe that they're eating tofu when they eat this low-fat dessert. It's creamy and rich, much like a cheesecake.

    1 cup Homemade Granola (page 222)
    2 teaspoons ground cinnamon
    safflower oil for pie pan
    1 pound (4 cakes) tofu
    1 cup Homemade Nonfat Yogurt (page 217)
    ¼ cup apple juice
    3 tablespoons mild-flavored honey
    2 teaspoons vanilla extract (more to taste)
    3 large ripe bananas
    ½ teaspoon nutmeg
    juice of 1½ lemons (more to taste)
    3 tablespoons whole wheat flour
    ½ cup fresh strawberries

Preheat the oven to 350 degrees.

Mix together the granola and 1 teaspoon cinnamon.

Brush a 9- or 10-inch pie pan or an 8-inch springform pan lightly with safflower oil and sprinkle the granola evenly over the bottom.

Blend together the tofu, yogurt, apple juice, honey, vanilla, 2 bananas, nutmeg, 1 teaspoon cinnamon, the juice of 1 lemon, and the whole wheat flour in a blender or food processor until completely smooth. Make sure there are no little chunks of tofu left unblended.

Pour into the prepared baking dish and bake in the preheated oven for 50 minutes, until the top is just beginning to brown. Remove from the oven and cool, then chill several hours.

Before serving, slice the remaining banana and toss with remaining lemon juice. Cut the strawberries in half, and decorate the top of the pie with the banana slices and strawberries.

DAY 6

BREAKFAST
>   Mixed Grains Muesli
>   Fresh Orange Juice

LUNCH
>   Gazpacho
>   Tabbouleh
>   Orange-Mint Sherbet

DINNER
>   Pizza
>   Tossed Green Salad (page 228)
>   Fresh Grapes

RECIPES

Mixed Grains Muesli
Serves 4

>   2½ cups water
>   ½ cup rolled or flaked oats
>   ½ cup flaked wheat or flaked triticale
>   2 tablespoons bran
>   1 teaspoon cinnamon or 1 stick cinnamon
>   ½ teaspoon freshly grated nutmeg
>   ¼ cup raisins
>   2 tablespoons wheat germ
>   1 tablespoon broken pecans
>   1 tart apple, grated
>   1 cup Sweet Yogurt Cereal Topping (page 202) (optional)

Bring the water to a rolling boil in a saucepan. Mix together the oats, wheat or triticale flakes, and the bran. Slowly pour into the boiling water while stirring. Add the cinnamon, nutmeg, and

raisins. Cover, reduce heat, and simmer 15 minutes until the
liquid is absorbed. Sprinkle the wheat germ, pecans, and grated
apple over the top and serve. If you wish, moisten each bowl
with not more than ¼ cup of the topping.

Gazpacho
Serves 6

    8 ripe tomatoes, peeled (see Note) and cut in chunks
    1 small onion, coarsely chopped
    1 carrot coarsely chopped
    ¾ bell pepper, coarsely chopped
    ¾ cucumber, peeled and coarsely chopped
    1 small hot pepper or hot banana pepper (optional)
    2 cloves garlic, peeled
    3 sprigs parsley
    ¼ cup chopped fresh basil or 1 tablespoon dried
    ½ teaspoon anise seeds (optional)
    1 cup water (more as necessary)
  ¼–½ cup lemon juice
    ¼ cup vinegar, plus more to taste
      freshly ground pepper to taste

FOR THE GARNISH
choice or combination of:
    1 cup cubed tofu
    2 ripe tomatoes, peeled (see Note) and minced
      the ¼ remaining cucumber, minced
      the ¼ remaining bell pepper, minced
    ½ cup grated carrot
    ¼ cup Homemade Nonfat Yogurt (page 217)
    2 tablespoons sunflower seeds
    ½ cup alfalfa or mung bean sprouts

In a blender or food processor, purée the vegetables, herbs,
anise seeds, water, lemon juice, and vinegar in batches until
smooth. Grind in black pepper to taste and chill for several
hours. Adjust seasonings, adding more lemon juice or vinegar as
desired.

Mix together the tofu, minced tomatoes, cucumbers, bell
peppers, and grated carrot in a small bowl. Place heaping spoon-

fuls of this mixture in each serving bowl and spoon in the soup. Top with a small dollop of yogurt, a sprinkling of sunflower seeds, and a small handful of sprouts. Serve chilled or at room temperature.

Note: To peel tomatoes, drop into boiling water for 20 seconds, drain, and run under cold water.

Tabbouleh
Serves 6

This is a delicious salad of cracked wheat and herbs. For a more intense flavor, make it a day early and allow it to sit overnight in the refrigerator. The cumin gives it a special lift.

½ cup lemon juice
½ cup vinegar
½ teaspoon dry mustard or Homemade Mustard Without Salt (page 211)
1 clove garlic, minced or put through a press
1 teaspoon ground cumin
1¼ cups water
1½ cups raw bulgur
1 cup cooked garbanzos (page 171)
2 tablespoons safflower oil
¾ cup minced fresh parsley
1 cup minced green onion
½ cucumber, peeled and diced
3 ripe tomatoes, diced
¼–½ cup chopped fresh mint (optional)
1 head romaine lettuce

Method 1: If you have time to make this a day in advance, mix together the lemon juice, vinegar, mustard, garlic, cumin, and water. Toss with the bulgur and the remaining ingredients, except the romaine lettuce, and refrigerate overnight or for several hours. If the bulgur is not completely submerged in liquid, add a little more water. Toss every so often to make sure all the bulgur is marinating evenly.

Method 2: If preparing and serving the tabbouleh the same day, bring the water to a boil and pur over the bulgur. Allow it to sit for 15 to 20 minutes. Mix together the lemon juice, vinegar, oil, garlic, mustard, and cumin and stir into the bulgur. Add the herbs, garbanzos, and vegetables and toss. Refrigerate for an hour or so.

For either method, line a salad bowl with the large outer leaves of the romaine and fill with the tabbouleh. Garnish with the smaller leaves, which you can stick into the salad in a circle and use as dippers.

Orange-Mint Sherbet
Serves 4 to 6

    4 cups orange juice (can be from unsweetened concentrate)
    ¼ cup chopped fresh mint

Blend together the orange juice and mint and freeze in a sorbettier (see page 160) or an ice cream freezer.

Pizza
Makes three 10-inch pies

You may be hooked on homemade pizza after you try this. The crusts can be made in advance and frozen for future meals—they take only about 25 minutes to thaw. The tomato sauce also can be made well in advance and frozen, or it can be kept in a covered container in the refrigerator for a few days.

    FOR THE CRUST
    2 tablespoons honey
    2 tablespoons active dry yeast
    1¼ cups lukewarm water
    3 tablespoons safflower oil, plus additional
    4 cups whole wheat flour
    corn meal

FOR THE TOMATO SAUCE

2 teaspoons safflower oil
1 onion, chopped
5 cloves garlic
3 pounds tomatoes, chopped
6 ounces unsalted tomato paste
1 bay leaf
pinch of cinnamon
1–2 teaspoons dried oregano, to taste
1 tablespoon chopped fresh basil or 1 teaspoon dried
1 teaspoon mild-flavored honey
freshly ground pepper

FOR THE TOFU CREAM SAUCE

½ pound (2 cakes) tofu
½ cup Homemade Nonfat Yogurt (page 217)
2 tablespoons sesame tahini
1 tablespoon lemon juice
pinch or two of nutmeg
pinch of cayenne pepper (optional)

ADDITIONAL TOPPINGS

1 bell pepper, sliced
1 onoin, sliced
1 cup sliced fresh mushrooms

Make the crust: In a large bowl, dissolve the honey and the yeast in the water. Let it sit 10 minutes, then stir in the 3 tablespoons safflower oil and begin stirring in the flour, 1 cup at a time. After you have stirred in 3 cups the dough should come away from the sides of the bowl. Place ½ cup flour on your kneading surface and scrape out the dough. Knead according to the directions on page 177, adding more flour as necessary. When the dough is smooth and elastic, oil your bowl, form the dough into a ball, and place in the bowl seam side up first, then seam side down. Let rise for 1 to 1½ hours until it has doubled in volume.

Punch down the dough and knead again for a few minutes. Divide into three equal pieces and roll out each piece to a thickness of about ¼ inch. Oil three 10-inch pizza pans and dust with corn meal. Place the dough on them and pinch a lip around the edge. At this point the crusts can be frozen or refrigerated until ready to use (cover tightly in plastic).

Start the tomato sauce: Heat the safflower oil and sauté the onion with half the garlic until the onion is tender. Add the tomatoes, tomato paste, and bay leaf and bring to a simmer. Simmer, uncovered, for 30 minutes. Add the additional garlic, the cinnamon, and the herbs and simmer for another 30 minutes or longer. Add the honey and ground pepper to taste.

Preheat the oven to 400 degrees. Prebake the crusts for 7 minutes. Remove from the heat and raise oven temperature to 450 degrees.

Make the tofu cream sauce: Place all tofu sauce ingredients in blender and blend until smooth.

Spread the tomato sauce over the crusts, then spread the tofu cream sauce over it.

Use any or all of the other toppings. Green peppers, onions, and mushrooms can be sprinkled on raw, or sautéed in 1 to 2 teaspoons safflower oil until slightly soft. Distribute them over the tofu cream sauce.

Bake in the hot oven for 10 minutes, or until the crust is brown and the pizzas smell deliciously ready.

DAY 7

BREAKFAST
> *Couscous with Fruit*
> *Half Grapefruit with Strawberries*

LUNCH
> *Split Pea Soup*
> *Corn on the Cob*
> *Herbed Triticale Bread (page 179) or Whole Wheat Sage*
> *and Onion Bread (page 180) (optional)*
> *Mixed Sprouts Salad*
> *Sliced Peaches*

DINNER
> *Artichokes with Low-Fat Tomato "Béarnaise"*
> *Tossed Green Salad (page 228)*
> *Herbed Triticale Bread (page 179) or Whole Wheat Sage*
> *and Onion Bread (page 180) with Mushroom Spread (page*
> *188)*
> *Italian Fruit Compote*

RECIPES

Couscous with Fruit
Serves 4

> 1 cup couscous
> 2 cups water
> ½ cup apple juice
> ¼ cup raisins
> 1 apple, cored and chopped
> 1 pear, cored and chopped
> ½–1 teaspoon ground cinnamon
> ½ teaspoon nutmeg

Place the couscous in a bowl and pour on the water. Heat the apple juice in a skillet and add the raisins, apple, and pear. Cook over medium heat until the fruit begins to soften, about 3 minutes. Add the spices and cook another 3 to 5 minutes.

After 10 minutes the couscous should be "cooked." Toss with the fruits over medium heat in the skillet just to heat through, and serve.

Split Pea Soup
Serves 6

    2 teaspoons safflower oil
    1 onion, chopped
    2–4 cloves garlic, to taste, minced or put through a press
    2 cups split peas
    2 carrots, sliced
    7 cups water
    1 teaspoon (or more) cumin and/or curry powder (optional)
    1 bay leaf
    2–4 tablespoons chopped fresh parsley
    freshly ground pepper
    lemon juice to taste

Heat the oil in a heavy-bottomed soup pot or Dutch oven and sauté the onion with half the garlic until the onion begins to soften. Add the split peas, carrots, water, optional curry or cumin (or both), and bay leaf and bring to a boil. Reduce heat, cover, and simmer for 30 minutes. Add the remaining garlic and cook another 30 minutes. Add the parsley and season to taste with plenty of black pepper and lemon juice.

Mixed Sprouts Salad
Serves 6

> 1 cup alfalfa sprouts
> 1 cup lentil sprouts
> 1 cup mung bean sprouts
> ½ cup chopped green onions
> 2 tablespoons sunflower seeds
> 1 cup diced peeled cucumber
> ½ cup diced green pepper
> 1–3 tablespoons chopped fresh herbs, such as basil, thyme, rosemary, marjoram, or dill, alone or in combination (optional)
> Yogurt Vinaigrette (page 195)
> 2 ripe tomatoes or 12 cherry tomatoes

Toss together all the ingredients except the tomatoes. Decorate the salad with tomatoes and serve, or chill and serve.

Artichokes with Low-Fat Tomato "Béarnaise"
Serves 4

> 4 artichokes
> 1 cup dry white wine
> 1 cup water
> 4 cloves garlic, but into thirds
> 1 slice of onion
> 1 bay leaf
> 1 sprig parsley
> juice of ½ lemon
> Low-Fat Tomato "Béarnaise" (page 206)

Trim the artichokes by cutting off the top third with a sharp knife and snipping off the spiny end of each leaf with kitchen shears (this sounds tedious, but it actually goes quickly). Cut the stems flush with the bottom of the artichoke.

Combine the dry white wine, water, garlic, onion, bay leaf, parsley, and lemon juice in a large Dutch oven. Place the artichokes in this mixture (stem end up) and bring to a simmer.

Cover and simmer 45 minutes, or until the leaves come away easily from the stems.

Serve hot, warm, room temperature, or chilled with the "béarnaise."

Italian Fruit Compote
Serves 6

> ¼ cup raisins or currants
> ½ cup apple juice
> 1 tart apple, diced
> 1 pear, diced
> 1 banana, sliced
> juice of ½ lemon
> 1 small bunch red grapes, halved
> 4 figs, dried or fresh, chopped

Soak the raisins or currants in the apple juice while you prepare the other fruit. Toss the diced apple, pear, and sliced banana with the lemon juice. Remove grape seeds if you want to take the time. Combine all the ingredients, including their soaking liquid, in a large glass bowl and chill until ready to serve.

DAY 8

BREAKFAST
> *Honeydew Smoothies*
> *Toasted Bread (pages 179–84) with Apple Spice Tofu*
> *Morning Spread (page 192)*

LUNCH
> *Brown Rice Salad*
> *Steamed Squash and Cauliflower*
> *Baked Apples*

DINNER
> *Vegetable Platter with Spinach Yogurt Spread*
> *Baked Sweet Potatoes with Lime Juice*
> *Yeasted Corn Bread (page 184)*
> *Watermelon Sherbet*

RECIPES

Honeydew Smoothies
Serves 4

These are mouth-watering, especially when the honeydew is very ripe. There is so much sweet liquid in the melon that it will blend up into a thick drink with no additional liquid. Ice is optional.

> 1 ripe honeydew
> crushed ice as desired
> 2 tablespoons chopped fresh mint (optional)

Remove the seeds and rind from the melon and blend until smooth. The drink will be very thick. Add crushed ice or mint if desired.

Brown Rice Salad
Serves 4 to 6

1 cup raw brown rice
1 green pepper, diced
1 sweet red pepper, if available, diced
4 radishes, sliced
½ cucumber, peeled and diced
3 talbespoons sunflower seeds
¼ cup Roasted Soybeans (page 221)
½ cup chopped fresh parsley
¼ cup chopped fresh basil, if available
4 green onions, chopped
1½ cups Low-Fat Vinaigrette (page 195) or Yogurt Vinaigrette (page 195)
leaf lettuce
2 tomatoes, sliced, or 10 cherry tomatoes
1 cup alfalfa sprouts
additional green onions and herbs for garnish (optional)
lemon wedges

Cook the rice according to the directions on page 169. Meanwhile prepare the vegetables and the vinaigrette.

When the rice is cooked, toss with the vinaigrette, peppers, radishes, cucumber, sunflower seeds, soybeans, herbs, and green onions. Chill for an hour or so. Line a platter or salad bowl with the lettuce leaves and fill with the salad. Garnish with the tomatoes, sprouts, additional green onions and herbs if you like, and lemon wedges, and serve.

Steamed Squash and Cauliflower
Serves 4

1 zucchini, sliced ½ inch thick
1 yellow squash, sliced ½ inch thick
½ head caluflower, broken into florets
herbs, such as thyme, rosemary, dill, marjoram, basil (optional)
lemon wedges

Steam the vegetables together for 10 minutes, or to taste. Toss with herbs, if you wish, and serve with lemon wedges on the side.

Baked Apples
Serves 4

> 4 tart apples
> ½ cup apple juice
> 2 tablespoons raisins
> cinnamon and nutmeg to taste
> safflower oil for baking dish
> ½ cup water

Preheat the oven to 350 degrees.

Core the apples by cutting a cone shape from the stem end down to the bottom, being careful not to cut through the bottom. Fill each cavity with a tablespoon of apple juice and 1½ teaspoons raisins. Add cinnamon and nutmeg to taste.

Place the apples in a lightly oiled baking dish, and pour in the remaining apple juice and the water. Bake in the preheated oven for 45 minutes, or until tender.

Vegetable Platter with Spinach Yogurt Spread
Serves 6 to 8

> 2 cups broccoli pieces
> 2 cups cauliflower pieces
> ½ pound carrots, cut in 3-inch sticks
> 1 medium zucchini, cut in 3-inch spears
> 1 medium yellow squash, cut in 3-inch spears
> ½ pint cherry tomatoes
> 10 radishes
> Spinach Yogurt Spread (page 190)

Steam the broccoli very briefly, just until bright green (after you see the steam escaping from the pan, count to 15 and drain). Arrange the vegetables in an attractive pattern on a platter, alternating colors and shapes. You might want to put the broccoli and cauliflower in the middle, like a flower, and surround it with alternating carrot, yellow squash, and zucchini spears, with cherry tomatoes and radishes dotting the arrangement here and there. Alternatively, put the spinach dip in the center and work around it.

Baked Sweet Potatoes with Lime Juice
Serves 4

You can use either sweet potatoes or yams for this. They both have such a deep, rich flavor of their own that they hardly need anything else. Lime juice is traditionally used in Latin American countries, where sweet potatoes are a staple.

    4 sweet potatoes
    2 large or 4 small limes

Preheat the oven to 425 degrees. Pierce the sweet potatoes several times with a fork and bake 40 to 50 minutes, or until thoroughly tender. Cut open and season to taste with lime juice.

Watermelon Sherbet
Serves 4 to 6

    4 cups watermelon pulp, seeds removed
    ¼ cup lime juice
    1 banana

Blend together the ingredients until smooth. Freeze in an ice cream maker or sorbettier.

DAY 9

BREAKFAST
> *Oatmeal with Apples, Spices, and Raisins (page 225)*
> *Fresh Orange Juice*

LUNCH
> *Buckwheat Noodle Salad with Hot and Sour Dressing*
> *Tomatoes Stuffed with Lentils*
> *Pineapple Boats*

DINNER
> *Baked Acorn Squash*
> *Bulgur-Spinach Salad with Poppy Seed Dressing*
> *Sliced Oranges*

RECIPES

Buckwheat Noodle Salad with Hot and Sour Dressing
Serves 4

> ½ pound buckwheat noodles
> 1 cup mung bean sprouts
> 1 small cucumber, peeled and coarsely grated
> 1 small zucchini, cut in matchsticks
> ½ cup Roasted Soybeans (page 221)
> 5 radishes, sliced
> 5 green onions, sliced
> 4–5 mushrooms, sliced
> 3 tablespoons chopped fresh coriander (cilantro)
> Hot and Sour Dressing (page 198)
> 1 head lettuce, leaves separated, washed, and dried

Bring a large pot of water to a boil and add the buckwheat noodles. Cook al dente, which should take about 4 to 5 minutes,

drain, and rinse with cold water. Toss with the remaining
ingredients, except the lettuce. Refrigerate for an hour or so, or
serve at once, in a bowl or on a platter lined with lettuce leaves.

Tomatoes Stuffed with Lentils

Serves 6

The lentils for this can be held in the refrigerator for up to 4
days. They freeze well.

> ¾ cup lentils, washed and picked over
> 1 small onion, chopped
> 2–3 cloves garlic, minced or put through a press
> 1 small carrot, minced
> 3½ cups water
> 1 bay leaf
> pinch or 2 of thyme
> 1 teaspoon of cumin
> ½ teaspoon chili powder
> freshly ground pepper
> 6 large, firm ripe tomatoes
> 3 tablespoons chopped fresh parsley
> 1 tablespoon finely grated or chopped lemon peel
> ½ cup Herbed Bread Crumbs (page 185) or whole wheat
>   bread crumbs
> safflower oil for baking dish

Combine the lentils, onion, garlic, carrots, water, bay leaf,
thyme, cumin, and chili powder in a large, heavy-bottomed saucepan, and bring to a boil. Cover, reduce heat, and cook 45 minutes
or until the lentils are tender. Grind in black pepper to taste.

Meanwhile, cut the tops off the tomatoes about ½ inch down
from the stem. Carefully scoop out the seeds and pulp and cut
out the inner flesh with a small sharp knife, leaving the shells of
the tomatoes intact. Chop the flesh which you removed and stir
into the lentils.

Drain the lentils and toss with the parsley and lemon peel.

Preheat the oven to 400 degrees.

Spoon the lentils into the tomatoes and top with the bread
crumbs. Place in a lightly oiled baking dish and bake 20 to 30
minutes, until the tomatoes are sizzling.

Pineapple Boats
Serves 6

> 1 large ripe pineapple
> 1 pint strawberries
> ½ pint blueberries
> 3 kiwis, peeled and cut into rounds
> 2 tablespoons chopped fresh mint

Cut the pineapple in half without removing the leaves. Use a grapefruit knife or a sharp stainless steel knife to cut out the fruit, leaving the skins intact (cut into the halved pineapple on the diagonal). Cut away the core and discard, and chop the pineapple. Toss with the strawberries and blueberries and return to the pineapple shells. Place these on a platter and surround with the excess fruit. Layer some of the beautiful light green kiwi across the top of the boats, and distribute the rest around the pineapples. Sprinkle with mint.

Baked Acorn Squash
Serves 4 to 6

> 2–3 acorn squash, cut in half lengthwise, seeds removed
> ground cinnamon to taste
> ¼–½ cup apple juice
> 2 apples, cut in rounds
> safflower oil for baking dish
> ½ cup water

Preheat the oven to 375 degrees.

Sprinkle the acorn squash with cinnamon and place a tablespoon of apple juice in each cavity. Layer the rounds of apple across the top of the acorn squash and place in a lightly oiled baking dish. Add ½ cup water to the dish, cover with foil or a lid, and bake in the preheated oven for 1 hour or until the squash is tender.

Bulgur-Spinach Salad with Poppy Seed Dressing
Serves 6

    1½ cups bulgur
    3 cups boiling water
    ½ pound spinach, washed and chopped
    4 ounces (1 cake) tofu, crumbled
    2 tablespoons sesame seeds
    1 tablespoon chopped fresh parsley
    1 tablespoon chopped fresh mint (optional)
    Poppy Seed Dressing (page 197)

Place the bulgur in a bowl and pour on the boiling water. Let sit 30 minutes, or until the water is absorbed and bulgur is soft. If the bulgur on top is not absorbing enough water, toss from time to time. Drain off excess water when the bulgur is tender. Toss with the remaining ingredients and chill until ready to serve.

DAY 10

BREAKFAST
> *Couscous with Fruit (page 254)*
> *Fresh Grapefruit Juice*

LUNCH
> *Cucumber Raita*
> *Curried Tofu and Vegetables*
> *Millet (page 169)*
> *Assorted Melon Balls*

DINNER
> *Cabbage with Apples*
> *Bulgur (page 170)*
> *Tossed Green Salad (page 228)*
> *Strawberries in Orange Juice*

RECIPES

Couscous with Fruit

Cook twice what you need, and use the excess (you'll need 1 cup) for making muffins tomorrow (see page 269).

Cucumber Raita
Serves 6

> 2 medium-size cucumbers
> ½ teaspoon dried coriander
> ½ teaspoon ground cumin
> ¼ teaspoon ground cardamom
> ½ cup Homemade Nonfat Yogurt (page 217)

Peel, seed, and finely chop the cucumbers. Add the spices to the yogurt. Toss all ingredients together.

266

Curried Tofu and Vegetables
Serves 4 to 6

Serve this curry over hot cooked millet. It goes well with Mixed
Fruit Chutney (page 216) on the side.

    2 teaspoons safflower oil
    1 onion, sliced
    1 clove garlic, minced or put through a press
    1 teaspoon grated fresh ginger or ½ teaspoon dried
    2–3 teaspoons curry powder
    ½ teaspoon cumin seeds
    ½ pound (2 cakes) tofu, diced
    ¼ cup white wine or apple juice
    1 medium carrot, sliced ¼ inch thick
    1 zucchini, sliced ¼ inch thick
    1 yellow squash, sliced ¼ inch thick
    2 tablespoons sunflower seeds
    3 tablespoons raisins
    ½ cup Homemade Nonfat Yogurt (page 217)
    1–2 tablespoons chopped fresh coriander (cilantro) (optional)

Heat the oil in a large, heavy-bottomed skillet and add the
onion, garlic, and ginger. Sauté, stirring for about 3 minutes,
until the onion begins to soften. Add the curry powder and
cumin seeds, the tofu, and the white wine or apple juice and
cook, stirring, for 3 to 5 minutes. Add the carrot and cook
another 5 minutes, then add the zucchini, yellow squash, sunflower seeds, and raisins. If the pan is dry, add a little water.
Cover and cook, stirring, for 5 to 10 minutes, until the squash is
crisp and tender. Transfer to a serving dish and toss with the
yogurt and, if you wish, coriander.

Assorted Melon Balls
Serves 4

    ½ ripe honeydew
    ½ ripe cantaloupe
    chopped fresh mint to taste

Scoop out melon balls with a melon baller and toss in a bowl
with the fresh mint. Chill until ready to serve.

Cabbage with Apples
Serves 4 to 6

>   2 teaspoons safflower oil
>   1 onion, sliced
>   ½ medium head red cabbage, shredded
>   2 tart apples, peeled and sliced
>   1 tablespoon raisins
>   3 tablespoons apple juice
>   3 tablespoons red wine vinegar
>   1 teaspoon cinnamon
>   ½ teaspoon allspice
>   ½ teaspoon ground cloves
>   ⅓ cup Homemade Nonfat Yogrut (page 217) (optional)

Heat the safflower oil in a large, heavy-bottomed skillet and sauté the onion until tender. Add the red cabbage and apples and sauté another 3 minutes, stirring. Add the raisins, apple juice, vinegar, cinnamon, allspice, and cloves and cook over medium heat, stirring from time to time, for about 5 to 10 minutes. Remove from the heat, let cool a moment, and stir in the yogurt if you like. (If the pan is too hot the yogurt will curdle.)

Strawberries in Orange Juice
Serves 6

>   2 pints strawberries, washed, hulled, and sliced
>   1½ cups orange juice
>   ½ teaspoon ground cinnamon
>   ¼ teaspoon ground cardamom

Toss together all the ingredients and chill.

DAY 11

BREAKFAST
Couscous Muffins with Apple Spice Tofu Morning Spread
Sliced Peaches

LUNCH
Mushroom and Barley Soup
Herbed Triticale Bread (page 179)
Tossed Green Salad (page 228)
Sliced Pears

DINNER
Kidney Beans with Corn and Pumpkin or Winter Squash
Coleslaw
Sliced Cantaloupe

RECIPES

Couscous Muffins with Apple Spice Tofu Morning Spread
Makes 12 muffins

2 tablespoons flax seeds
¼ cup water
1 cup Couscous with Fruit (page 254)
½ cup whole wheat flour
1 teaspoon ground cinnamon
½ teaspoon nutmeg
1 tablespoon mild-flavored honey
1 tablespoon safflower oil, plus additional for muffin tins
2 tablespoons Homemade Nonfat Yogurt (page 217)
Apple Spice Tofu Morning Spread (page 192)

Preheat the oven to 375 degrees.
Grind the flax seeds in a blender or spice mill. Pour water over them. Allow to sit for 10 minutes.

269

Mix together the couscous with the flour, cinnamon, and nutmeg. Mix together the honey, safflower oil, and yogurt. Stir the flax seeds with soaking water into the grain mixture. Mix together well and spoon into lightly oiled muffin tins.

Bake for 20 minutes in the preheated oven. Serve with tofu spread.

Mushroom and Barley Soup

Serves 6

> 2 teaspoons safflower oil
> 1 large onion, chopped
> 2 cloves garlic, minced or put through a press
> ½ pound mushrooms, rinsed and sliced
> 1 green pepper, chopped
> ¼ cup dry white wine
> ⅓ cup soy flakes
> 1½ cups barley
> ½ teaspoon dried thyme (more to taste)
> ¼–½ teaspoon dried rosemary
> 2 quarts water
> 2 tablespoons sherry
> freshly grated nutmeg (optional)
> ¼ cup chopped fresh parsley
> freshly ground pepper

Heat the safflower oil in a large, heavy-bottomed soup pot or Dutch oven and sauté the onion with 1 clove garlic until the onion is tender. Add the mushrooms, green pepper, and wine and continue to sauté another 5 minutes, stirring, until the mushrooms become tender and aromatic. Add the remaining garlic, the soy flakes, barley, thyme, and rosemary, stir together for a couple of minutes over a medium flame, and add the water. Bring to a boil, reduce the heat, and cover. Simmer 45 to 60 minutes, checking from time to time to make sure that there is enough liquid. (The soup should be quite thick.) Add the sherry and, if you wish, a little nutmeg. Just before serving, stir in the parsley and season to taste with a generous amount of black pepper.

Kidney Beans with Corn and Pumpkin or Winter Squash
Serves 6 to 8

This is a succotash of sorts, made with kidney beans. (Lima beans or lentils may be substituted.) The down-to-earth flavors and the colors of the beans, corn, and pumpkin are very appealing. Paprika gives added flavor.

    2 teaspoons safflower oil
    1 medium onion, thinly sliced
    1–2 cloves garlic, to taste, minced or put through a press
    2 tablespoons mild paprika
    ¼ cup red wine
    kernels from 2 large ears of corn
    1 pound pumpkin or winter squash (such as butternut),
        seeds removed, peeled, and diced
    1 pound tomatoes, peeled (see Note), seeded, and chopped
    ½–1 teaspoon dried oregano, to taste
    8 ounces beans or lentils (page 171)
    freshly ground pepper to taste
    chopped fresh parsley
    lemon juice to taste (optional)

Heat the safflower oil in a large, heavy-bottomed skillet and add the onions and garlic. Sauté over medium heat until the onion begins to soften, and add the paprika. Cook a minute, stirring, and add the red wine. Continue to cook, stirring, until the onions are tender. Add the corn, pumpkin or squash, tomatoes, and oregano, and cover. Simmer 15 to 20 minutes or until the squash is cooked through and beginning to fall apart. Stir in the cooked beans, toss to distribute the heat evenly, and season to taste with pepper and parsley. Add lemon juice, if you wish.

Note: To peel tomatoes, drop into boiling water for 20 seconds, drain, and run under cold water.

Coleslaw
Serves 6 to 8

4 cups shredded cabbage
½ cup grated onion
juice of 1 lemon
½ cup vinegar
2 tablespoons mild-flavored honey
2 tablespoons apple juice
1½ tablespoons chopped fresh dill or 2 teaspoons dried
freshly ground pepper to taste
½ cup water or Homemade Nonfat Yogurt (page 217)

Toss together the cabbage and onion. Mix together the lemon juice, vinegar, honey, apple juice, dill, pepper, and water or yogurt. Toss with the cabbage. Serve chilled or at room temperature.

DAY 12

BREAKFAST

>Fresh Orange Juice
>Sliced Bananas
>Toasted Bread (pages 179–84) with Apple Spice Tofu
>Morning Spread (page 192)

LUNCH

>Potato-Tomato Soup
>Herbed Triticale Bread (page 179) or Whole Wheat Sage
>and Onion Bread (page 180)
>Spinach Salad (page 227)
>Baked Pears

DINNER

>Pasta with Vegetables
>Tossed Green Salad (pages 228) with Parsley Vinaigrette
>   (page 196)
>Bread (pages 179–84) with Choice of Spreads (pages
>   186–92)
>Red or Green Grapes

RECIPES

Potato-Tomato Soup
Serves 6 to 8

  1 teaspoon safflower oil
  1 large onion, chopped
  2 cloves garlic, minced or put through a press
  3 tablespoons dry white wine
  1 pound russet potatoes, scrubbed and sliced
  1 carrot, sliced
  1½ pound tomatoes, peeled (see Note) and sliced
  ½ teaspoon dried thyme
  6 cups water
  1 teaspoon dried sweet basil or 1 tablespoon chopped fresh
  2 tablespoons red wine
  freshly ground pepper to taste

Heat the safflower oil in a large, heavy-bottomed soup pot or Dutch oven and sauté the onion with 1 clove of garlic until the onion begins to soften. Add the white wine, potatoes, carrot, tomatoes, and thyme and continue to sauté for about 3 minutes. Add the water and bring to a boil. Cover, reduce heat, and simmer 30 minutes. Add the basil and the second clove of garlic and simmer another 15 minutes or until the potatoes fall apart. Purée half the soup and return to the pot. Add the red wine, season to taste with freshly ground pepper, and serve.

Note: To peel tomatoes, drop into boiling water for 20 seconds, drain, and run under cold water.

Baked Pears
Serves 6

  6 ripe but firm pears
  2 tablespoons apple juice
  1 tablespoon vanilla extract
  cinnamon
  nutmeg

Preheat the oven to 325 degrees.
Core the pears by cutting out a cone shape from the stem

down, so that you leave the bottom intact. Combine the apple juice and vanilla and drizzle into the pears. Sprinkle on cinnamon and nutmeg.

Place in a lightly oiled baking dish and bake 45 minutes, or until soft.

Pasta with Vegetables
Serves 6

The cracked roasted soybeans give a nice contrast of textures and flavors to the dish.

1 medium carrot, sliced ¼ inch thick
1 zucchini, sliced ¼ inch thick
1 yellow squash, sliced ¼ inch thick
1 pound eggless whole wheat fettucine
½ pound tomatoes, peeled (see Note), seeded, and chopped
½ cup chopped fresh parsley
2–3 tablespoons chopped fresh herbs, such as basil, oregano, thyme, marjoram, rosemary, sage (if available)
1–2 teaspoons finely grated lemon
¼ cup Roasted Soybeans (page 221), cracked in a blender
freshly ground pepper to taste

Begin steaming the carrots. After 5 minutes add the zucchini and squash and continue to steam for 10 minutes. Remove from the heat and refresh under cold water. Vegetables should be crisp-tender and bright.

Bring a large pot of water to a boil and cook the fettucine al dente (that is, until firm to the bite). Spoon into a warm serving dish using a slotted spoon or deep-fry skimmer (you can also drain in a colander, but you will lose some of the heat). Toss immediately with the steamed vegetables, tomatoes, herbs, grated lemon, cracked roasted soybeans, the pepper, and serve.

Note: To peel tomatoes, drop into boiling water for 20 seconds, drain, and run under cold water.

DAY 13

BREAKFAST
> *Homemade Granola (page 222) with Sweet Yogurt Cereal Topping (page 202)*
> *Fresh Orange Juice*

LUNCH
> *Fruit Soup*
> *Bread (pages 179–84)*
> *Millet Raisin Pudding*

DINNER
> *Spaghetti Squash with Tofu-Tomato Sauce*
> *Marinated Cucumber Salad*
> *Mixed Fruit Ice*

RECIPES

Fruit Soup
Serves 6 to 8

> 1 pound peaches, peeled (see Note) and sliced
> 1 pound plums, sliced
> 1 pound nectarines, sliced
> ½ pound apples, peeled, cored, and sliced
> 1 banana, peeled and sliced
> 4 cups water
> juice of 1 lemon
> 2 tablespoons tapioca
> ½ cup Homemade Nonfat Yogurt (page 217)

Combine the fruit and water and bring to a boil. Reduce heat, cover, and cook 15 minutes. Add the lemon juice and tapioca and continue to cook until the mixture thickens. Serve each portion topped with a tablespoon of yogurt. Serve either hot or chilled.

Note: To peel peaches, drop into boiling water, count to 10, drain, and run under cold water. Skins will slip off easily.

Millet Raisin Pudding
Serves 6

>1 cup raw millet
>2 cups water
>2 teaspoons vanilla extract
>¼ cup instant soy milk (such as Fearn)
>¼ cup mild-flavored honey
>½ teaspoon cinnamon
>½ cup raisins
>safflower oil for baking dish

Preheat the oven to 350 degrees. Combine the millet and water in a saucepan and bring to a boil. Drain off the water into a blender and blend with the vanilla, soy milk, honey, and cinnamon until you have a homogeneous mixture. Stir back into the millet and toss with the raisins.

Oil a 2-quart baking dish and fill with the millet mixture. Cover and bake in the preheated oven for 30 to 40 minutes, until the liquid is absorbed.

Spaghetti Squash with Tofu-Tomato Sauce
Serves 6

Spaghetti squash (also known as banana squash) is a recently popular vegetable that is now fairly common. The large squashes look something like oval melons. They have a delicious, fibrous pulp that makes spaghetti-like strands when cooked and scraped from the yellow outer rind. The strands can be served with almost any sauce that accompanies pasta. They also make a nice salad marinated in a low-fat vinaigrette.

2 small or 1 large spaghetti squash
2 teaspoons safflower oil
1 small onion, minced
1 small carrot, minced
3 cloves garlic, minced
½ pound (2 cakes) tofu, crumbled
3 pounds fresh tomatoes, seeded and chopped or puréed
one 6-ounce can unsalted tomato paste
pinch of cinnamon
2 teaspoons fresh basil or 1 teaspoon dried
1 teaspoon dried oregano
freshly ground pepper to taste
2 tablespoons chopped fresh parsley
¼ cup herbed or toasted bread crumbs

Spaghetti squash can be baked whole in a 350-degree oven for 1 hour, or steamed on top of the stove for 30 minutes. To steam, place the whole squash in a large pot in a small amount of water or on a steamer and steam for 30 minutes, until tender when pierced with a fork. Remove from the heat and cut in half lengthwise. Remove the seeds and inner pulp (not the spaghetti strands) by scraping crosswise. Then scoop out the spaghetti strands by scooping lengthwise with a spoon. Set this aside, covered.

Begin the sauce while the spaghetti squash is steaming. Heat the safflower oil and sauté the onion and carrot with 1 clove of the garlic until the onion is tender. Add the tofu and mash it with the back of a spoon, then add the tomatoes, tomato paste, and remaining garlic. Bring to a simmer and cook, covered, for 30 minutes. Add a pinch of cinnamon, the basil, oregano, and pepper to taste, and cook uncovered another 10 minutes.

Spoon the spaghetti squash into a warm serving dish, top with the tomato sauce, garnish with parsley and bread crumbs, and serve.

Marinated Cucumber Salad
Serves 6

    ½ cup vinegar
    1 clove garlic, minced or put through a press
    ¼ cup lemon juice
    1 tablespoon chopped fresh dill or 1 teaspoon dried
    1 teaspoon dill seeds
    freshly ground pepper
    1 cup water
    1½ pounds cucumbers, peeled, if waxed, and thinly sliced
    1 white or red onion, sliced thin

Mix together the vinegar, garlic, lemon juice, dill, dill seeds, pepper, and water and toss with the cucumbers and onions. Chill. Serve with a slotted spoon to eliminate as much liquid as possible.

Mixed Fruit Ice
Serves 4 to 6

    2 cups fresh pineapple
    2 bananas
    1 cup strawberries
    2 peaches, peeled and sliced
    1 cup orange juice
    1 cup Homemade Nonfat Yogurt (page 217)
    1 teaspoon vanilla extract

Blend the ingredients together and freeze in an ice cream freezer or sorbettier.

Note: If you have leftover Fruit Soup from lunch, you could substitute that for the fruit, put it through a blender, and freeze in a sorbettier or ice cream freezer.

DAY 14

BREAKFAST
> *Mixed Grains Muesli (page 248)*
> *Half Grapefruit*

LUNCH
> *Grated Zucchini Casserole with Eggplant Sauce*
> *Vegetable Platter with Spinach Yogurt Spread (page 260)*
> *Citrus Salad*

DINNER
> *Crudité Salad*
> *Bulgur Pilaf*
> *Apple Crisp*

RECIPES

Grated Zucchini Casserole with Eggplant Sauce
Serves 6

> 2 large eggplants
> 2 pounds zucchini, grated
> ½ teaspoon dried thyme or 1 teaspoon fresh
> freshly ground pepper to taste
> 2 teaspoons safflower oil, plus additional for baking dish
> 3 cloves garlic
> 1 teaspoon ground cumin (optional)
> juice of 1 lemon (or to taste)
> 3 tablespoons minced fresh coriander (cilantro) (optional)
> ½ cup minced fresh parsley
> ¼ cup Roasted Soybeans (page 221), cracked in a blender
> ½ pint cherry tomatoes

Cook the eggplant according to the directions on page 175. Remove from the oven and turn the heat down to 325 degrees.

When the eggplant is cool enough to handle, scoop out the pulp and chop fine.

Heat a large, heavy-bottomed skillet over a medium flame and cook the zucchini in its own liquid for 5 minutes, or until tender. Toss with the thyme and freshly ground pepper to taste, and remove from the heat. Place in a lightly oiled 2- or 3-quart casserole and set aside.

Heat the 2 teaspoons safflower oil in the same skillet in which you sautéed the zucchini and add the garlic and eggplant. Sauté, stirring, for 5 to 10 minutes, until the eggplant is thoroughly tender and aromatic. Add the cumin (optional), the lemon juice, and plenty of pepper. Stir in the fresh coriander (optional) and half the parsley, and remove from the heat.

Spoon the eggplant onto the squash and top with the soybeans and the remaining parsley. Place cherry tomatoes around the edge of the baking dish for decoration. Serve at once, or heat for 5 minutes and serve.

Citrus Salad
Serves 6

> 3 oranges
> 1 grapefruit
> 1 tablespoon chopped fresh mint

Peel the oranges and grapefruit by cutting the peel away in a spiral, with a knife angled into the fruit slightly so that you trim away the white pith at the same time. Slice crosswise into ¼-inch slices. Arrange on a platter and garnish with the mint. Chill until ready to serve.

Crudité Salad
Serves 6

3–4 medium potatoes
Low-Fat Vinaigrette (page 195)
freshly ground pepper
1 tablespoon minced green onion, both white and green parts
1 tablespoon chopped fresh parsley
½ pound fresh green beans, trimmed
1 large carrot, grated
6 radishes, cut in half
4 ripe tomatoes, sliced in wedges, or ½ pint cherry tomatoes
1 cucumber, scored with a fork or peeled, then sliced
1 cup alfalfa sprouts
1 head Boston or red tip lettuce, leaves separated, washed, and drained
fresh herbs for garnish (such as basil, thyme, marjoram, dill)

Wash the potatoes (without removing the peel) and steam for about 20 minutes, until tender. Remove from the heat and slice immediately into a bowl. Pour on ¼ cup of the vinaigrette, then toss gently with the pepper, green onion, and parsley. Cover and chill.

Steam the green beans no more than 5 minutes, until crisp-tender, and refresh under cold water.

If you are serving the salad on a platter: Toss the green beans, carrots, radishes, tomatoes, cucumber, and sprouts individually with portions of the dressing. Line the platter with the lettuce leaves. Place the green beans in the center, surround them with potatoes interspersed with tomato wedges or cherry tomatoes, mounds of carrots, and radishes. Circle with rounds of cucumbers and clumps of sprouts. Garnish with fresh herbs.

If serving in a bowl: Make a similar arrangement, or toss everything except the lettuce together with the vinaigrette. Use the lettuce to line the bowl. Garnish with fresh herbs.

Bulgur Pilaf
Serves 6

  1½ cups bulgur
  3 cups water
  1 teaspoon safflower oil
  1 onion, chopped
  2 tablespoons sunflower seeds
  1 teaspoon crushed cumin seeds
  3 tablespoons raisins or currants
  ¼–½ teaspoon ground cardamom
  1 tablespoon apple concentrate or tamarind concentrate
    (available in Middle Eastern markets) (optional)

Place the bulgur in a bowl. Bring the water to a boil and pour over the bulgur. Allow it to sit for 30 minutes.

Meanwhile heat the oil in a large, heavy-bottomed skillet and sauté the onion with the sunflower seeds until tender. Add the cumin seeds, raisins or currants, and cardamom and sauté another 2 minutes. Remove from the heat, toss with the bulgur and the apple or tamarind concentrate (if you wish), and serve.

Apple Crisp
Serves 6 to 8

  2 tablespoons safflower oil, plus additional for baking pan
  2 tablespoons apple concentrate or mild-flavored honey
  2½ cups rolled or flaked oats
  ¼ cup whole wheat pastry flour
  2 teaspoons ground cinnamon
  1 teaspoon allspice
  ½ teaspoon nutmeg
  10 tart apples or cooking apples
  juice of 1 lemon
  2 teaspoons vanilla extract
  ½ cup apple or orange juice
  ½ cup Homemade Nonfat Yogurt (page 217)

Preheat the oven to 325 degrees.

Combine the oil with the honey or apple concentrate and mix together with the oats, pastry flour, and half the spices.

Slice the apples and toss with the lemon juice, vanilla, and remaining spices.

Brush a 2- or 3-quart oblong pan lightly with safflower oil. Spread half the apple mixture over this. Top with half the oat mixture. Spread the remaining apples over this and top with the remaining oat mixture. Pour on the apple or orange juice and bake 45 minutes in the preheated oven, or until crisp.

Garnish each serving with a tablespoon of yogurt.

DAY 15

BREAKFAST
> *Cream of Wheat with Raisins and Cinnamon (page 239)*
> *Fresh Blueberries*

LUNCH
> *Roasted Soybean, Sprouts, and Tomato Sandwich*
> *Tossed Green Salad (page 228)*
> *Oranges with Mint*

DINNER
> *Marinated Mushrooms*
> *Black Bean Chalupas*
> *Papaya with Lime*

RECIPES

Roasted Soybean, Sprouts, and Tomato Sandwich
Makes 1 sandwich

> 2 thin slices or 1 thick slice Herbed Triticale Bread (page 179) or Whole Wheat Sage and Onion Bread (page 180)
> Homemade Mustard Without Salt (page 211), to taste
> 1 tablespoons White Bean Spread (page 186) or Mushroom Spread (page 188) (optional)
> 2–3 slices ripe tomatoe
> 2 tablespoons alfalfa sprouts
> 1 tablespoon Roasted Soybeans (page 221), cracked in a blender
> vinegar or Low-Fat Vinaigrette (page 195) to taste

Spread bread with mustard and, if desired, the bean or mushroom spread. Top with sliced tomato, sprouts, and cracked roasted soybeans. Douse with vinegar or vinaigrette.

Oranges with Mint
Serves 4 to 6

>3 oranges, peeled, cut in rounds, with outer white membranes trimmed away
>2 tablespoons chopped fresh mint

Toss together and chill until ready to serve.

Marinated Mushrooms
Serves 6

>1 pound fresh mushrooms
>1½ cups water
>1½ cups cider vinegar
>4 whole cloves
>4 whole peppercorns
>¼ teaspoon mustard seeds
>½-inch stick of cinnamon
>pinch of dried rosemary
>1 bay leaf
>1 tablespoon safflower oil
>½ teaspoon dried basil
>½ teaspoon dried oregano
>¼ teaspoon dried thyme
>¼ cup chopped fresh parsley
>1 clove garlic, minced or put through a press
>freshly ground pepper
>leaf or romaine lettuce leaves, washed and dried
>1 tablespoon chopped fresh herbs, such as parsley, thyme, dill, chives, rosemary, oregano, or marjoram
>radishes
>cherry tomatoes

Wash the mushrooms and trim the stems. If they are very large, cut in half. Place in an enameled or stainless steel pot with the water, vinegar, cloves, peppercorns, mustard seeds, cinnamon, rosemary, and bay leaf. Bring to a boil, reduce heat, and simmer (covered) for 5 minutes. Turn off the heat and allow the mixture to sit for an hour or two.

Drain and rinse the mushrooms and toss with the safflower oil, herbs, and garlic. Add freshly ground pepper to taste and set aside for several hours, either in the refrigerator or at room temperature.

Line a platter or salad bowl with the lettuce and top with the mushrooms. Garnish with additional herbs, radishes, and cherry tomatoes.

Black Bean Chalupas
Serves 6 to 8

These are great for parties—it's fun to put together a chalupa, and the attractive ingredients make a buffet appear lavish. The various flavors and textures are terrific.

FOR THE BLACK BEANS
1 teaspoon safflower oil
1 onion, chopped
4 cloves garlic, minced or put through a press (more to taste)
1 pound black beans (pinto beans may be substituted), washed, picked over, and soaked
1 bell pepper, chopped, or 2 jalapeños, cut in half, seeds removed
6 cups water
1 tablespoon ground cumin (more to taste)
1 tablespoon chili powder (more to taste)
2 tablespoons choppled fresh coriander (cilantro) (more to taste)

FOR THE SALSA
3 tomatoes, chopped
¼ cup finely minced onion
2 very hot, fresh chilies, seeded and minced (serrano)
3 tablespoons chopped fresh coriander (cilantro)
4 tablespoons vinegar
¼ cup water

FOR THE REST OF THE CHALUPAS

12 corn tortillas
1 cup alfalfa sprouts
1 cup lentil sprouts
¼ cup sunflower seeds
½ cup finely chopped green onions
1 cup Homemade Nonfat Yogurt (page 217)
chopped fresh parsley or coriander (cilantro)
½ cup Low-Fat Vinaigrette (page 195) or plain vinegar
   (optional)

Cook the beans: Heat the safflower oil in a large, heavy-bottomed soup pot, Dutch oven, or bean pot and sauté the onion with 1 clove of garlic until the onion is tender. Add the beans, bell pepper or jalapeños, water, cumin, chili powder, and remaining garlic. Bring to a boil, reduce heat, cover, and simmer 2 hours or until tender. Add the fresh coriander and more garlic (to taste) halfway through the cooking.

When the beans are tender and aromatic, remove from the heat. Drain off and retain approximately ¾ of the liquid. Purée the beans in a food processor or a blender, or mash them using a potato masher or wooden spoon. The mixture should still have some texture. Moisten as desired with the cooking liquid. Taste and add more cumin, chili, or garlic as needed. Transfer to a serving dish.

While the beans are cooking, make the tortillas into chalupa crisps: preheat the oven to 250 degrees and bake the tortillas for 15 minutes until crisp—be careful that you do not burn them.

Make the salsa: Mix together the salsa ingredients and transfer to a decorative bowl.

For the rest of the chalupas: Place the remaining ingredients in individual bowls. Then place all the ingredients on a buffet. Party guests can assemble their own chalupas by spreading a generous amount of the black beans over the chalupa crisp, then topping with sprouts, a dollop of yogurt, salsa, a sprinkling of sunflower seeds, green onions, herbs, and a little vinaigrette or plain vinegar.

Papaya with Lime
Serves 4 to 6

    2 medium or large papayas, or 3 small ones
    2–3 limes

Cut the papayas in half, remove the seeds, peel, and slice. Squeeze on lime juice. Serve chilled or at room temperature.

DAY 16

BREAKFAST

> *Honeydew Smoothies (page 278)*
> *Toasted Bread (pages 179–84) with Apple Spice Tofu*
> *Morning Spread (page 192)*

LUNCH

> *Gazpacho Salad*
> *A Big Pot of Beans*
> *Bread (pages 179–84) such as Yeasted Corn Bread (page 184), or Corn Tortillas (page 185)*
> *Mixed Fruit Ice (page 275)*

DINNER

> *Vegetable Paella with Leftover Beans*
> *Marinated Cucumber Salad (page 279)*
> *Pineapple with Mint (page 234)*

RECIPES

Gazpacho Salad
Serves 6

> 3 cups peeled (see Note), seeded, and diced tomatoes
> 2 cucumbers, peeled, seeded, and diced
> 1 large red onion, poached 3 minutes and diced
> 2 bell peppers, diced
> 3 tablespoons wine vinegar
> Low-Fat Vinaigrette (page 195) or Yogurt Vinaigrette (page 195), with 2 extra cloves of garlic (extra garlic optional)
> 2 cups whole wheat bread crumbs
> 3 green onions, minced
> ½ cup chopped fresh parsley

In separate bowls, place the tomatoes, cucumbers, and onion. Add the green peppers to each bowl and toss with 1 tablespoon vinegar in each. Allow this to sit while you prepare the vinaigrette.

To assemble the salad, spread a fourth of the bread crumbs on the bottom of a glass bowl. Cover with a third of the onion mixture. Top this with a third of the tomatoes, and cover these with a third of the cucumbers. Pour on a fourth of the dressing, and repeat the layers. End with a layer of the bread crumbs, and pour on the remaining dressing. Sprinkle with green onions and parsley, cover, and chill until ready to serve.

Note: To peel tomatoes, drop into boiling water for 20 seconds, drain, and run under cold water.

A Big Pot of Beans
Serves 6 to 8

> 1 cup pinto beans, washed, picked over, and soaked
> ½ cup kidney beans, washed, picked over, and soaked
> ½ cup lima beans, washed, picked over, and soaked
> ½ cup garbanzos, washed, picked over, and soaked
> 2 onions, chopped
> 1 green pepper, chopped
> 6 cloves garlic, minced
> 1 bay leaf
> 2 sprigs parsley

Soak all the beans and cook with the onions, pepper, garlic, and herbs according to the directions on pages 171–73.

Vegetable Paella with Leftover Beans
Serves 8

- 1½ cups brown rice
- 3 cups water
- 2 teaspoons safflower oil, plus additional for sweet red pepper
- 2 onions, thinly sliced
- 4 cloves garlic, minced or put through a press
- 3 green peppers, seeded and sliced
- ¼ cup dry white wine
- 3 tomatoes, peeled (see Note) and sliced
- 1½ cups leftover cooked beans (any kind, or a mixture; garbanzos work especially well)
- 1 teaspoon Spanish saffron, if available
- 1 large bay leaf
- freshly ground pepper to taste
- 1 sweet red pepper, if available
- 1 cup fresh peas, steamed until bright green, or 1 cup frozen peas, thawed

Combine the rice and 1½ cups water in a saucepan and bring to a boil. Reduce heat, cover, and cook 20 to 30 minutes until the liquid is absorbed. The rice will be not quite cooked.

Heat the safflower oil in a large, heavy-bottomed skillet, paella pan, or wok, and sauté the onions with 2 cloves of the garlic until they start to become tender. Add the green peppers, wine, and remaining garlic and continue to sauté until the green peppers begin to soften (about 3 minutes). Add the tomatoes, rice, remaining water, cooked beans, saffron, and bay leaf and bring to a boil. Cover and cook 15 to 30 minutes until the liquid is absorbed and the rice is tender. Grind in plenty of black pepper.

While the paella is cooking, heat the broiler. Brush the red pepper with oil and place under the broiler, turning often, until it is uniformly charred. Remove from the heat and run under cold water. Remove the charred skin, cut in half, and remove the seeds and membranes. Now cut it in thin strips.

Add the peas to the top of the paella without stirring, and garnish with the red peppers. Cover and let heat 5 minutes, adding more liquid if necessary, and serve.

Note: To peel tomatoes, drop into boiling water for 20 seconds, drain, and run under cold water.

DAY 17

BREAKFAST
Rye-Oatmeal Bread with Anise and Raisins (page 182)
Apple Spice Tofu Morning Spread (page 192)
Sliced Melon

LUNCH
Acorn Squash Stuffed with Curried Millet and Fruit
Tossed Green Salad (page 228)
Frozen Banana Ice (page 242)

DINNER
White Bean Salad
Steamed Green Beans, Zucchini, or Broccoli
Herbed Triticale Bread (page 179) or Whole Wheat Sage
    and Onion Bread (page 180)
Tomatoes with Herbs
Cream of Wheat Delight

RECIPES

Acorn Squash Stuffed with Curried Millet and Fruit
Serves 6

2 apples, peeled, cored, and diced
2 pears, peeled, cored, and diced
juice of 1 lemon
1 cup apple juice
1 teaspoon curry powder (more to taste)
½ teaspoon allspice
¼ teaspoon ground cloves
3 tablespoons raisins
1 tablespoon sunflower seeds
1½ cups cooked millet (¾ cup raw; see page 169)
3 large acorn squash, halved, seeds removed
safflower oil for baking dish

Preheat the oven to 375 degrees.

Toss the apples and pears with the lemon juice.

Heat 2 tablespoons of the apple juice in a heavy-bottomed skillet and add the curry powder, allspice, ground cloves, apples, pears, raisins, and sunflower seeds. Cook, stirring, for 3 minutes. Remove from the heat and mix with the millet. Fill the acorn squash with this mixture, piling in as much as you can, and place in a lightly oiled baking dish. Moisten the stuffed squash by drizzling about 2 tablespoons apple juice over each. Place ½ cup water in the baking dish, cover with foil or a lid, and bake in the preheated oven for 45 to 60 minutes, until the squash is tender.

White Bean Salad
Serves 6 to 8

> 2 cups white beans, washed, picked over, and soaked
> 6 cups water
> 1 onion, chopped
> 3 cloves garlic, minced or put through a press
> 1 bay leaf
> 2 sprigs parsley
> 1 sprig fresh thyme or ¼ teaspoon dried
> 1 bell pepper, chopped
> 1 sweet red pepper, chopped, if available
> 4 green onions, chopped
> ½ cup chopped fresh parsley, or a combination of parsley, basil, marjoram, dill, and thyme
> 4 radishes, sliced
> 2 cups Low-Fat Vinaigrette (page 195)
> leaf lettuce, washed and dried
> 2 sliced tomatoes or 10 cherry tomatoes
> additional herbs for garnish (optional)

Cook the beans in the 6 cups water along with the onion, garlic, bay leaf, parsley sprigs, and thyme, according to the directions for Savory Beans on page 172.

When the beans are tender, drain, retaining the liquid. (You can use this liquid instead of water in the vinaigrette.) Toss the beans with the peppers, green onions, herbs, radishes, and vinaigrette. Refrigerate in a covered container for an hour or more.

Line a bowl or platter with the lettuce leaves and fill them with the beans. Garnish with tomatoes and additional herbs, if you wish, and serve.

Tomatoes with Herbs
Serves 6

3 ripe tomatoes, sliced
2 tablespoons chopped fresh herbs, such as basil, marjoram, parsley, or thyme
1 clove garlic, minced or put through a press (optional)
2 tablespoons wine vinegar or cider vinegar
¼ cup alfalfa sprouts (optional)

Place the tomatoes on a plate and sprinkle on the herbs. Mix the garlic with the vinegar. If you are using sprouts, place little clumps on top of the tomatoes. Drizzle on the vinegar and serve.

Cream of Wheat Delight
Serves 6

Cream of Wheat cereal takes on a new dimension here.

3 cups orange juice
2–3 tablespoons black cherry concentrate
½ cup non-instant farina, or Cream of Wheat
2 cups hulled strawberries
juice of ½ lemon
1 cup Homemade Nonfat Yogurt (page 217)
1 cup additional strawberries, sliced
thin strips of orange zest

Combine the orange juice and black cherry concentrate in a 1- or 2-quart saucepan and bring to a boil. Slowly add the farina or Cream of Wheat in a thin stream, stirring constantly. Cook, while stirring, until thick and smooth (about 8 to 10 minutes). Pour into a large bowl and whip with a wire whisk or electric beater until light and fluffy. Fold in the 2 cups strawberries, lemon juice, and yogurt. Chill.

Serve garnished with sliced strawberries and grated orange rind.

DAY 18

BREAKFAST
> *Seven-Grain Cereal*
> *Fresh Orange Juice*

LUNCH
> *Cauliflower Salad*
> *Carrot Soup*
> *Bread (pages 179–84)*
> *Fruit Salad*

DINNER
> *Couscous Casserole*
> *Steamed Brussels Sprouts with a sauce of your choice (pages 200–207)*
> *Tossed Green Salad (page 228)*
> *Raspberry Ice*

RECIPES

Seven-Grain Cereal
Serves 4

These cereals are easy to find in health food stores. (The Health Valley Company makes a good one.) There are several brands; not all have seven grains (some have more, some less), but most provide a nice balance of textures and flavors and are quite filling. You can add raisins, fruit, or spices as you desire.

> 2½ cups water
> 1 cup seven-grain cereal
> up to 3 tablespoons raisins, or 1 cup diced fruit, as you wish
> ½–1 teaspoon cinnamon
> ¼–½ teaspoon allspice
> ¼–½ teaspoon nutmeg

Bring the water to a boil and slowly pour in the cereal. Add raisins or diced fruit and spices, cover, and cook 30 minutes until the liquid is absorbed. For the fruit to remain crunchy, wait until the last 10 minutes to add it. Serve with Sweet Yogurt Cereal Topping (page 202).

Cauliflower Salad
Serves 4 to 6

1 large head caulfilower, broken into smaller pieces
1 Bermuda onion, sliced thin
¼ cup chopped fresh parsley
2 tablespoons other chopped fresh herbs, such as basil, thyme, marjoram, dill, if available
1½ cups Low-Fat Vinaigrette (page 195), with double amount of mustard
2 tomatoes, sliced, or 10 cherry tomatoes
radishes
green onions
alfalfa sprouts

Steam the cauliflower and Bermuda onion together for 5 to 10 minutes, to taste. Drain and refresh under cold water. Toss with the herbs and vinaigrette, and chill until ready to eat. This also can be served warm.

Transfer to a salad bowl and garnish with combination of tomatoes, radishes, green onions, and sprouts.

Carrot Soup
Serves 6

2½ pounds carrots, scrubbed and sliced
1 large potato, peeled and diced
1 onion, chopped
4 cups water
½ teaspoon dried thyme (more to taste)
1½ cups Homemade Nonfat Yogurt (page 217)
1 tablespoon lime juice (more to taste)
freshly ground pepper
3 tablespoons sunflower seeds

Combine the carrots, potato, onion, water, and thyme in a soup pot or Dutch oven and bring to a simmer. Cover and cook 40 minutes. Purée in a blender or through a food mill and return to the pot. Stir in the yogurt, and season to taste with lime juice and freshly ground pepper. Heat through but do not boil, or the yogurt will curdle. Garnish with sunflower seeds, and serve hot or cold.

Fruit Salad
Serves 6

> 2 peaches, peeled and sliced
> 2 plums, sliced
> 1 apple, cored and sliced
> 1 orange, peeled and chopped
> 1 cup green grapes
> juice of 1 lime
> fresh mint

Toss together the fruit and the lime juice. Chill until ready to serve. Garnish with fresh mint.

Couscous Casserole
Serves 6 to 8

> 2 cups broccoli florets
> 4 ripe tomatoes, peeled (see Note)
> 1 teaspoon safflower oil, plus additional for baking dish
> 1 onion, diced
> 1 clove garlic, minced or put through a press
> 1 teaspoon grated fresh ginger
> ½ pound (2 cakes) tofu, diced
> 1 teaspoon paprika
> 2 tablespoons vinegar
> 1 tablespoon mild-flavored honey
> 3 cups cooked couscous (1½ cups raw; see page 170)

Steam the broccoli 5 minutes, drain, and refresh under cold water. Set aside.

Slice two of the tomatoes and set aside. Purée the rest in a blender or food processor.

Heat the 1 teaspoon oil in a heavy-bottomed skillet and add the onion and garlic. Sauté until the onion begins to soften. Add the ginger, tofu, tomato purée, paprika, vinegar, and honey. Simmer this mixture together over a medium flame, uncovered, for 10 to 15 minutes.

Preheat the oven to 325 degrees.

Toss together the tomato-tofu mixture and the couscous. Fill a lightly oiled 2- or 3-quart baking dish with this mixture. Decorate the top with alternating rows of sliced tomatoes and broccoli. Cover with foil or a lid and heat in the oven for 20 to 30 minutes.

Note: To peel tomatoes, drop into boiling water for 20 seconds, drain, and run under cold water.

Raspberry Ice
Serves 4 to 6

> 4 cups unsweetened frozen raspberries
> juice of 1 lemon
> 2 tablespoons black cherry concentrate or mild-flavored honey
> fresh mint and/or fresh raspberries for garnish

Blend together the raspberries, lemon juice, and black cherry concentrate or honey in a blender or food processor until smooth. Freeze in a sorbettier or ice cream freezer. Garnish with fresh mint or fresh raspberries and serve.

DAY 19

BREAKFAST
> *Homemade Granola (page 222) with Sweet Yogurt Cereal Topping (page 202)*
> *Sliced Peaches*

LUNCH
> *Cucumber-Potato Salad*
> *Steamed Snow Peas*
> *Strawberries with Yogurt*

DINNER
> *Beet Salad*
> *Soybean-Grains Casserole*
> *Steamed Asparagus*
> *Deep-Dish Peach Pie*

RECIPES

Cucumber-Potato Salad
Serves 4 to 6

> 2 pounds new or boiling potatoes, scrubbed and unpeeled
> 1 bunch green onions, minced
> ¼ cup snipped fresh chives
> 1½ cups Yogurt Vinaigrette (page 195)
> 1 cucumber, peeled and thinly sliced
> 2 tablespoons minced fresh dill
> freshly ground pepper

Steam the potatoes about 20 to 25 minutes until just tender. Drain, rinse under cold water, and slice thin. Toss with the green onions, chives, vinaigrette, cucumber, dill, and freshly ground pepper to taste. Refrigerate until ready to serve, or serve warm.

Steamed Snow Peas
Serves 4

> 1 pound snow peas, trimmed, with strings removed
> fresh lemon juice or herbs, as desired

Steam the snow peas 5 minutes until crisp-tender. Drain and serve with lemon juice or herbs to taste.

Strawberries with Yogurt
Serves 1

> ½ cup sliced strawberries
> 2 tablespoons Homemade Nonfat Yogurt (page 217)

Place sliced strawberries in a bowl and top with a dollop of yogurt.

Beet Salad
Serves 4 to 6

> 1½ pounds whole beets, scrubbed
> 2 cups water
> ½ cup tarragon or white wine vinegar
> 2 tablespoons safflower oil
> 1 teaspoon caraway seeds, ground in a spice mill or blender (optional)
> 4 whole cloves
> 1 clove garlic, cut in thirds
> juice of 1 lemon
> 2 tablespoons snipped fresh dill or 1 teaspoon dried
> 1 tablespoon chopped fresh parsley

Trim the beets and place them on a steamer above approximately 2 cups water. Bring the water to a boil, cover, and steam beets 30 minutes or until crisp and tender all the way through (this may take longer for large beets). Remove from the steamer and run under cold water until cool enough to handle. Peel off the skin and add the skin to the steaming water. Add the vinegar, safflower oil, caraway seeds (if you like), whole cloves, and garlic and bring to a boil. Boil 15 minutes or until the mixture is reduced by half. Meanwhile, slice the beets ¼ inch thick (or thinner).

Strain the liquid and add the lemon juice. Toss with the beets, dill, and parsley. Chill. Serve with a slotted spoon to eliminate as much liquid as possible.

Soybean-Grains Casserole
Serves 6 to 8

>2 teaspoons safflower oil, plus additional for casserole
>1 onion, chopped
>2–3 cloves garlic, minced or put through a press
>1 cup sliced mushrooms (optional)
>½ teaspon dried thyme
>1 tablespoon dry white wine
>5 cups chopped tomatoes
>1 small carrot, grated or minced
>6-ounce can unsalted tomato paste
>1 teaspoon dried oregano
>1 teaspoon dried basil or 1 tablespoon chopped fresh
>pinch of cinnamon
>freshly ground pepper to taste
>3 zucchini, sliced ¼ inch thick
>2 cups cooked brown rice or bulgur, or a combination (see pages 169 and 170)
>2 cups cooked soybeans or soy flakes (⅔ cup raw; see page 174)
>½ cup whole wheat bread crumbs
>2 tablespoons chopped fresh parsley

Heat the 2 teaspoons safflower oil in a heavy-bottomed sauce-pan and sauté the onion and 1 clove of the garlic until the onion begins to soften. Add the mushrooms (if you like), thyme, and white wine. Continue to sauté, stirring, until the mushrooms are aromatic (about 5 minutes). Add the tomatoes, carrot, tomato paste, oregano, and dried basil, if using it, and bring to a simmer. Simmer, uncovered, for 30 minutes, stirring occasionally. Add the cinnamon, pepper, and fresh basil. Cook 5 more minutes and remove from the heat.

Meanwhile, steam the zucchini 5 minutes. Refresh under cold water, and set aside.

Preheat the oven to 325 degrees. Brush a 2- or 3-quart casserole lightly with safflower oil.

Mix together the cooked grains and soybeans with a cup of the tomato sauce. Spread this mixture in the baking dish. Top with the zucchini, and pour on the remaining tomato sauce. Sprinkle bread crumbs over the top and bake 30 minutes in the preheated oven. Sprinkle on the parsley and serve.

Deep-Dish Peach Pie
Serves 8 to 10

> Yeasted Pie Crust (page 181)
> 5 cups peaches, peeled and sliced
> 2 tablespoons apple concentrate
> 1½ teaspoons ground cinnamon
> ½ teaspoon freshly grated nutmeg
> 1½ teaspoons vanilla extract
> 1 tablespoon cornstarch
> 1 tablespoon lemon juice

Make the pie dough according to the recipe. Roll out and retain a portion for the lattice. Line a 2-quart baking dish with the bottom crust. Prebake 5 minutes at 400 degrees. Turn the oven up to 425 degrees.

Mix together the peaches, apple concentrate, cinnamon, nutmeg, and vanilla in a bowl. Dissolve the cornstarch in the lemon juice and stir it into the peaches. Turn into the pie crust.

Roll out the section you retained for the lattic and cut ¾- or 1-inch-wide strips. Weave a lattice over the peaches.

Bake 10 minutes at 425 degrees, then turn the heat down to 350 degrees. Bake another 30 minutes, or until the top browns. Remove from the heat and cool. Serve warm or cool.

DAY 20

BREAKFAST
> Half Grapefruit
> Toasted Bread (pages 179–84) with Apple Spice Tofu
> Morning Spread (page 192)

LUNCH
> Coleslaw with Cucumbers
> Hoppin' John (Mixed Beans and Grains)
> Bread (pages 179–84)
> Fresh Pineapple

DINNER
> Green Peppers Stuffed with Hoppin' John
> Steamed Turnips and Brussels Sprouts
> Tossed Green Salad (page 228)
> Citrus Salad (page 281)

RECIPES

Coleslaw with Cucumbers
Serves 6 to 8

> ½ medium head green cabbage, shredded
> ½ pound carrots, scrubbed and grated
> ½ cup finely grated onion
> ¼ cup plus 3 tablespoons vinegar
> 2 tablespoons mild-flavored honey
> ¾ cup Homemade Nonfat Yogurt (page 217)
> 1 medium cucumber, peeled and thinly sliced
> 1 tablespoon fresh dill or 1 teaspoon dried

Toss together the cabbage, carrots, and onion.

Mix together ¼ cup vinegar, the honey, and the yogurt, and toss with the vegetables.

Toss the sliced cucumber with 3 tablespoons vinegar and the dill. Add ¼ cup water to the cucumber if not serving the salad right away, and let it marinate for an hour or so in the refrigerator. Drain the cucumbers and top the coleslaw with them just before serving.

Hoppin' John (Mixed Beans and Grains)
Serves 6

For directions on soaking the various beans in this recipe, see page 171.

> ½ cup raw wheat berries
> 1 cup brown rice
> ¾ cup pinto beans, washed, picked over, and soaked
> ¾ cup lima beans, washed, picked over, and soaked
> ¾ cup red kidney beans, washed, picked over, and soaked
> ¾ cup black-eyed peas, washed, picked over, and soaked
> 1 large onion, chopped
> 5 cloves garlic, minced or put through a press
> 1 bell pepper, seeded and chopped, or 2 jalapeños, cut in half, seeds removed
> 3 sprigs fresh coriander (cilantro) (more to taste)
> 1 bay leaf
> 1 teaspoon dried thyme
> 6 cups water
> freshly ground pepper

Cook the wheat berries and the rice separately, according to the general cooking directions on pages 169–70.

Cook all the beans together with the onion, garlic, pepper, coriander, bay leaf, and thyme in the 6 cups water, according to the directions for Savory Beans on page 172. Adjust seasonings, adding garlic, black pepper, and other herbs or spices of your choosing. Stir in the rice, and serve. Use the leftovers for Green Peppers Stuffed with Hoppin' John (page 306), or freeze.

Green Peppers Stuffed with Hoppin' John
Serves 4 to 6

    4–6 medium or large bell peppers
    3–4 cups leftover Hoppin' John (page 305)
    safflower oil for baking dish
    1½ cups alfalfa sprouts
    2 tablespoons chopped fresh herbs, such as parsley, basil,
        thyme, rosemary, marjoram

Preheat the oven to 375 degrees. Cut the tops off the peppers about ½ inch down from the stems. Carefully scoop out the seeds and inner membranes. Fill with the Hoppin' John (about ½ to ¾ cup in each pepper). Place the caps back on and place in a lightly oiled baking dish.

Bake in the preheated oven for 30 minutes or until tender. Remove the caps again and garnish with sprouts and herbs. Serve with caps either on or off.

DAY 21

BREAKFAST
> *Fruit-Filled Coffee Cake Braid*
> *Fresh Orange Juice*

LUNCH
> *Cucumber-Yogurt Soup*
> *Bread (pages 179–84) with White Bean Spread (page 186)*
> *or Mushroom Spread (page 188)*
> *Strawberry Sherbet*

DINNER
> *Sautéed Eggplant*
> *Brown Rice (page 169) or Couscous (page 170)*
> *Tossed Green Salad (page 228)*
> *Berries and Cherries in Cantaloupe*

RECIPES

Fruit-Filled Coffee Cake Braid
Makes 1 large briaded coffee cake

FOR THE DOUGH
1 tablespoon active dry yeast
½ cup warm water
1 tablespoon malt syrup
½ cup orange juice (fresh or from concentrate)
¼ cup soy powder
1 tablespoon grated orange rind
2 cups unbleached white flour
2 tablespoons safflower oil, plus additional
1 teaspoon ground cinnamon
2 cups whole wheat flour

FOR THE FILLING

2 peaches, peeled and sliced
2 plums, sliced
2 apples, peeled and sliced
1 banana, sliced
1 cup seedless grapes
1 teaspoon vanilla extract
1 teaspoon ground cinnamon
½ cup unsweetened fruit spread (page 168)

FOR THE GLAZE

2 tablespoons apple concentrate
¼ cup water

Make the dough: Dissolve the yeast in the warm water in a large bowl and stir in the malt syrup. Heat the orange juice to lukewarm and stir into the yeast mixture. Stir in the soy powder, orange rind, and unbleached white flour. Stir approximately 100 times, cover with plastic or a damp towel, and set in a warm place to rise for 1 hour.

When the hour is up and the sponge is bubbling, fold in the oil and 1 teaspoon cinnamon. Then fold in the whole wheat flour, a cup at a time, and turn onto a lightly floured board. Knead for at least 10 minutes, adding unbleached flour if necessary, until smooth and elastic. Form into a ball, oil the bowl, and place the dough in it seam side up, then seam side down. Cover and let rise 1 hour.

Make the filling: Mix together all the filling ingredients except the unsweetened fruit spread.

Punch down the dough, turn out onto your work surface, and roll it into a rectangle about 16 inches long and 12 inches wide. Spread with unsweetened fruit spread. Spread the filling down the center third of the rectangle. Now, using a sharp knife, cut the dough on either side into 1-inch strips pointed in a downward angle. Fold these strips in over the filling, alternating sides so that you are weaving one over the other like a braid. When you get to the end, pinch the braids over the lower end. Carefully transfer the coffee cake to a lightly oiled baking sheet. Let rise for 40 minutes. Preheat the oven to 350 degrees.

Bake in the preheated oven for 30 to 40 minutes, until golden brown. While it is baking, mix together the apple concentrate and ¼ cup water. Simmer over a medium flame. When you remove the coffee cake from the oven, glaze it with this mixture. Serve warm.

Cucumber-Yogurt Soup

Serves 6

> 3 cucumbers, peeled and coarsely chopped
> 1 quart Homemade Nonfat Yogurt (page 217)
> 1 tablespoon chopped fresh dill or 1 teaspoon dried
> 1 teaspoon dill seeds
> 1 clove garlic (more to taste)
> 1 teaspoon chopped fresh mint (optional)
> juice and grated frind of 1–2 lemons, to taste
> cucumber slices
> lemon slices
> alfalfa sprouts

Blend the chopped cucumbers, yogurt, dill, dill seeds, garlic, mint (if you like), and lemon juice and rind together in a blender or food processor until smooth. Chill and serve. Garnish each bowl with thin slices of cucumber and lemon and a small amount of sprouts.

Strawberry Sherbet

Serves 4 to 6

> 2 pints strawberries, hulled
> 1 tablespoon black cherry concentrate
> 3 tablespoons lemon juice
> fresh mint

Blend together the strawberries, black cherry concentrate, and lemon juice in a blender or food processor until smooth. Freeze in a sorbettier or ice cream freezer. Garnish with fresh mint.

Sautéed Eggplant
Serves 6 to 8

>   2 eggplants, cut in half lengthwise
>   2 teaspoons safflower oil, plus additional for baking sheet
>   1 onion, sliced
>   2 cloves garlic, minced or put through a press
>   1 green pepper, seeded and diced
>   4 ounces (1 cake) tofu, diced or crumbled (optional)
>   3 tablespoons dry white wine
>   3 tablespoons sunflower seeds
>   2 tomatoes, peeled (see Note) and sliced
>   2 teaspoons chopped fresh basil or 1 teaspoon dried
>   1 tablespoon chopped fresh parsley
>   ½ teaspoon allspice or cumin (optional)
>   ½ cup whole wheat bread crumbs
>   1 tablespoon lime juice (more to taste)
>   freshly ground pepper to taste

Preheat the oven to 450 degrees. Score the eggplants down to but not through the skin, and place on a baking sheet that is brushed lightly with safflower oil. Bake 20 minutes, until the eggplant is soft. Remove from the heat. When the eggplant is cool enough to handle, scoop out from the skins, and dice.

Heat the 2 teaspoons safflower oil in a heavy-bottomed skillet and sauté the onion, garlic, and green pepper until the onion begins to soften. Add the diced eggplant, the optional tofu, and the white wine and continue to sauté another 5 minutes. Add the sunflower seeds, tomatoes, herbs, allspice or cumin (if you wish), and bread crumbs. Continue to sauté over medium heat, stirring from time to time, for another 10 to 15 minutes. Add lime juice to taste and grind in plenty of pepper. Serve with brown rice, couscous, or another grain of your choice.

Note: To peel tomatoes, drop into boiling water for 20 seconds, drain, and run under cold water.

Berries and Cherries in Cantaloupe
Serves 4 to 6

  1 cup blueberries
  ½ cup raspberries
  1 cup pitted cherries, cut in half
  juice of 1 lime
  2–3 small cantaloupes, cut in half, seeds removed
  lime wedges
  fresh mint

Mix together the berries and cherries and toss with the lime juice. Fill the cantaloupe halves with the berries. Garnish with lime wedges and fresh mint. Serve chilled.

APPENDIX
SELECTED
BIBILIOGRAPHY
INDEX

Appendix. Effects of Stress Management Training and Dietary Changes in Treating Coronary Heart Disease*

The roles of both emotional stress and diet have long been suspected in the pathogenesis of ischemic heart disease (IHD).[1-2] Some emotions and behaviors are associated with IHD in a variety of populations; these include intense anxiety, depression, feelings of helplessness, and "Type A behavior," characterized by ambitiousness, competitiveness, impatience, and a sense of time urgency.[3-7] Biobehavioral techniques such as meditation, yoga, and progressive relaxation may elicit what Benson has termed the "relaxation response," which may reduce cardiovascular risk factors such as blood pressure[8-12] and plasma cholesterol[13-14] independent of dietary changes.

The evidence linking elevated lipids, particularly plasma cholesterol, to the development of IHD is well established.[15-19] Studies of vegan subgroups in this country have revealed lower plasma cholesterol, LDL, VLDL, and triglyceride levels, a higher HDL/LDL ratio, and lower blood pressure (BP) when compared with matched controls from the Framingham study; as the intake of animal products increased, the plasma cholesterol rose.[20-21] Case reports have suggested that changing to a vegan diet may reduce frequency of angina.[22]

We report the results of a randomized, controlled study to determine if a combination of training in stress management and an essentially vegan diet may produce short-term improvements in cardiovascular status in patients with IHD.

*Reprint of our cardiovascular research findings.

METHODS

Patient Selection

We audited all patient records (1977–1980) in the files of the nuclear cardiology and cardiac catheterization laboratories at St. Luke's Episcopal Hospital, the Methodist Hospital, and the Kelsey-Seybold Clinic, as well as the entire office records of two groups of cardiologists. We selected patients (ages forty-five to seventy-five) who had evidence of IHD: (1) greater than 50 percent stenosis in one or more major coronary arteries by cardiac catheterization; or (2) positive exercise radionuclide ventriculography, defined as a resting ejection fraction that fails to rise more than 5 percent with exercise and/or with regional wall motion abnormalities during exercise.[23] We excluded patients for any of the following reasons: resting ejection fraction less than 40 percent, cardiomyopathy, myocardial infarction (MI) or changes in cardiac medications within the preceding six months, carcinoma, cerebral vascular accident (CVA), psychosis, or previous coronary artery bypass surgery unless there was angiographically documented evidence of graft occlusion.

Using these criteria, 125 patients were eligible. Each was sent a letter describing the intervention (which began six weeks later) and a statement of informed consent. Fifty-one patients volunteered and were pre-tested during August 1980. Three patients were found to have a resting ejection fraction less than 40 percent and were excluded. The remaining 48 were randomly assigned to the experimental and control groups (24 patients each), using random number tables in a balanced randomization. During the study, one patient withdrew from each group (before post-testing), and their results are excluded from all analyses.

From this group of 48 volunteers, we randomly selected 19 experimental and 17 control patients to measure blood pressure reactivity to a series of tasks, some stressful. Due to scheduling and measurement problems, we excluded data from 4 experimental and 2 control patients, leaving 15 patients in each subgroup.

Study Design

The experimental group participated in a program of stress management training and dietary changes from September 3–27, 1980, while the control group continued their routine activities at work and home. Patients in the experimental group were housed together in a rural environment in order to maximize compliance to the intervention.

Appendix

The project staff prepared and served all meals at this site and trained the patients in stress management. Patients were required to consume only the food and beverages that were served to them; this was further reinforced by the relative inaccessibility of other food. Aerobic exercise (jogging, swimming, etc.) was not a formal component of this intervention.

Both groups were retested on all pre-intervention measures between September 27 and October 13, following the exact pre-intervention protocols. All tests were conducted at the Texas Medical Center in Houston. Technicians who processed the data and physicians who interpreted the results were blinded to patient identity, testing time (pre- or post-intervention), and group membership (experimental or control). The protocol was approved by the Human Subjects Committees of Baylor College of Medicine, St. Luke's Episcopal Hospital, and the Kelsey-Seybold Clinic.

Dependent Variables

EXERCISE RADIONUCLIDE VENTRICULOGRAPHY

The protocol for exercise radionuclide ventriculography has been described in detail in other publications.[24] Our protocol differed only slightly: we discontinued all medications for twelve hours prior to testing, and we tested patients in a sitting rather than in a supine position. In brief, 30 mCi of ^{99m}Tc-Pertechnetate was injected into an antecubital vein twenty minutes after injection of 6 mg stannous pyrophosphate to label red blood cells. All radioactive emissions were collected with the patient in the 45° sitting position using the Ohio Nuclear System 420/550 MOBILE Scintillation Camera. A 30° RAO resting gated image and a 45° resting LAO gated image were collected for 2½ minutes each. Electrocardiographic gating was employed by a computer to organize the acquired data into a series of images that span an average cardiac cycle. Images were displayed in rapid sequence as an endless-loop flicker-free movie so that wall motion could be evaluated. Globular ventricular function was assessed by determination of the ejection fraction, which is calculated from the ratio of the radioactive emissions (counts) after background correction collected from the left ventricle in end-diastole (ED) minus end-systolic (ES) counts to end-diastolic counts (ED), or (ED − ES)/ED. Blood pressure was obtained in the right arm brachial artery using the Infrasonde (Sphygmetrics) audible BP cuff utilizing an electronic transducer. After resting measurements were completed, the patient pedaled a bicycle ergometer at a load of 300 kpm/min (approximately 50-W) and this load was increased in 100 kpm increments in three-minute stages until stopping. After an initial thirty-second period to reset the R-R interval which was accepted by the computer, sequential LAO images were recorded during the remaining 2½ minutes of each stress period. Heart rate and BP were recorded at three-minute intervals in order to calculate the rate-pressure product. Reasons for stopping exercise included: exhaustion, severe chest pain, shortness of breath, attainment of maximum heart rate, ECG changes (ST displacement of 2 mm or more if flat or downsloping, or if J point is depressed 2 mm or more and return to baseline is 80 msec or longer), complex ventricular arrhythmias, systolic BP > 250 or diastolic BP > 140 mmHg or BP falling with increasing exercise. Three nuclear cardiologists reached a consensus on global ejection fraction and regional wall motion by viewing each patient's pre- and post-intervention study together as a random A/B comparison.

BLOOD PRESSURE RESPONSIVENESS TO STRESS
We took serial blood pressure readings from the right arm using appropriately sized cuffs with an embedded microphone linked to an electro-sphygmomanometer (Narco PE 300, programmed cuff inflation and deflation) and recorded on a Honeywell polygraph. After the patient was comfortably seated in the laboratory, the first BP reading was recorded after a three-minute resting period (trial #1, Figures A-1 and A-2). The patient then was presented with a standard set of stimuli, some stressful, including a series of six 0.25-second, 71-decibel tones or white noise (orienting response, trial #2), reaction tasks following a series of flashing lights preceded by ten-second tones (conditioning, trial #3), and a series of similar tones and lights without reaction time (extinction, trial #4).[25] Patients were then given difficult arithmetic problems or sentence construction tasks shown them on slides for thirty seconds each. BP was recorded before the first slide (trial #5), during the second slide (trial #6), and after the third slide (trial #7). After a one-minute rest (trial #8) the patients were then given a structured interview to assess and provoke Type A behavior, and BP was recorded during questions to assess the following characteristics: ambitiousness (trial #9), competitiveness (trial #10), and time urgency (trial #s 11 and 12).[26] After a five-minute rest, a final BP was measured (trial #13).

OTHER MEASUREMENTS
Plasma lipids were drawn after a 14-hour fast during which nothing but water was ingested. Blood was analyzed under laboratory

conditions standardized for the Lipid Research Clinics.[27] Angina frequency, smoking history, and medication usage were determined by questionnaire.

Intervention

STRESS MANAGEMENT TRAINING

Stress management techniques were taught and practiced five hours per day; this time was divided equally among the different techniques, in the order presented below. Each technique was presented as having the common purpose of increasing a patient's sense of relaxation, concentration, and awareness of internal states in order to retrain physiologic responsiveness to emotional stress.[14,28] Techniques included the following:

1. Stretching/relaxation exercises: Patients were taught simple, nonaerobic stretching exercises. They were advised to stretch slowly and gently and were carefully monitored to avoid injury or strain. Patients were directed to focus their attention on the areas being stretched and while resting to concentrate on their breathing. At the end of each class, each patient was instructed to progressively tense and relax muscle groups sequentially from feet to head, ending with a meditation (described below).[29]

2. Meditation: Each patient was asked to sit in a comfortable position and to breathe slowly and deeply while focusing his attention on his breathing, returning to it when attention wandered.[14-15,30-31]

3. Applied meditation (visualization): Each class began with a lecture on basic physiology and anatomy of the cardiovascular system and the pathophysiology of IHD to aid in constructing and maintaining a mental image. Following the lecture, each patient was instructed to meditate, as described above. After several minutes of meditation, each patient was asked to visualize his heart and coronary arteries, referring whenever necessary to drawings based on prior coronary angiography. With eyes closed, each patient was asked to visualize the atherosclerotic plaques being removed from the coronary arteries, using an image of his choice. Each class ended with the patients visualizing themselves as healthy, doing an activity which they enjoyed when they were without the physical limitations of IHD.[32]

4. Environment: The primary reason for housing patients together in a rural environment was to ensure compliance to the intervention. Approximately half the patients reported that the investigative setting contributed to their perceived reduction in stress, but the others said that it was more stressful for them to be away from their work, home, and family and to be living in close quarters with a new group of people.

Appendix

DIET

Patients were served a vegan diet (devoid of animal products) except for minimal amounts of nonfat yogurt. Also excluded were added salt, sugar, alcohol, and caffeine. They were served fresh fruits and vegetables, whole grains, legumes, tubers, and soybean products. The diet was verified for nutritional adequacy, with an average daily intake of 1400 calories, 325 mg sodium and 5.2 mg cholesterol. Particular attention was given to making the food attractive and appetizing. Daily classes were given in food purchasing, preparation, and nutrition.

Statistical Analysis

To compare the experimental and control groups at pre-intervention, we used Student's t-test (two tailed) on the interval data and Fisher's exact probability test on the categorical measures. To assess whether the experimental group improved relative to the control group post-intervention, we conducted analyses of covariance[33] on all interval data; the values of pre-intervention dependent measures were the covariates for the post-intervention measures. The ejection fraction response data were further analyzed using a three-way analysis of variance; the factors were (1) group (experimental vs. control), (2) time (pre- vs. post-intervention), and (3) condition (rest vs. maximal exercise).[34] Blood pressure responsiveness was analyzed, using a two-way analysis of variance (group x time). Group data are expressed as mean ± the standard error of the mean (S.E.M.).

RESULTS

Baseline Characteristics

There were no statistically significant pre-intervention differences (P > 0.05) between the experimental and control groups in age, sex, previous myocardial infarction, or previous coronary bypass surgery (Table 1). Also, there were no significant pre-intervention differences in any of the reported measures, with the exception of serum HDL, which was slightly higher in the experimental group (Table 2). Eighteen patients in the experimental and 21 patients in the control group had prior coronary angiography; they averaged 1.8 and 2.4 occluded arteries ≥ 50% (P > 0.05). In the experimental group, 7 had one-vessel, 7 had two-vessel, and 4 had three-vessel disease; in the control group, 6 had one-vessel, 8 had two-vessel, and 7 had three-vessel disease.

Table 1: Characteristics of Patients at Entry into Trial

Characteristics	Experimental Group	Control Group	Significance
	(n = 23)	(n = 23)	
Age (years)	58.3 ± 1.3	60.0 ± 1.6	§NS
Males	17	19	NS
Previous myocardial infarction	9	7	NS
Previous coronary bypass surgery	1	1	NS

Age is presented as mean ± S.E.M.; values in parentheses are ranges.
§§Not significant (P > 0.05, Student's t-test).

Exercise Tolerance

In the experimental group, total duration of exercise (bicycle ergometry) increased 44 percent (F = 20.1, P < 0.001), and total work performed increased 55 percent (F = 16.0, P < 0.0001), whereas the control group was essentially unchanged in both parameters (Table 3). Both groups achieved approximately the same rate-pressure products (systolic blood pressure x heart rate at peak exercise) post-intervention as pre-intervention, but the experimental group performed at a much higher workload before achieving the pre-intervention rate-pressure product (Table 3). Resting heart rate did not change significantly in either group.

Plasma Lipids

Changes in plasma lipids are outlined in Table 2. Overall, the experimental group showed a 20.5 percent reduction in plasma cholesterol (22 of 23 patients had reductions, even though most were not hyperlipidemic), while the control group did not change (F = 19.6, P < 0.0001). Triglycerides also were significantly reduced in the experimental group, but not in the control group (F = 6.5, P < 0.01). While HDL decreased in the experimental group, the total cholesterol/HDL ratio showed no significant differences between the groups.

Frequency of Angina

In the experimental group, the reported frequency of angina episodes per week decreased from 10.1 ± 2.0 pre-intervention, to 1.6 ± 0.5 after 2 weeks of the intervention, to 0.9 to 0.3 post-intervention.

Table 2: Plasma Lipid and Lipoprotein Levels

Measurement	Period	Experimental Group	Control Group	Significance*
Plasma cholesterol	pre	229.0 ± 9.3	220.9 ± 10.3	P < 0.0001
(mg/dl)	post	182.0 ± 8.4	215.2 ± 9.7	
Plasma triglycerides	pre	188.9 ± 21.2	245.8 ± 67.7	P < 0.01
(mg/dl)	post	159.7 ± 13.1	248.0 ± 48.2	
HDL (mg/dl)	pre	47.1 ± 2.2	38.8 ± 3.3	P < 0.0001
	post	39.2 ± 1.8	38.2 ± 3.0	
Total cholesterol/HDL	pre	5.06 ± 0.35	6.34 ± 0.50	§NS
	post	4.65 ± 0.22	6.27 ± 0.54	

Data are presented as mean ± S.E.M.
*Changes in the experimental group were compared with changes in the control group using an analysis of covariance: the pre-intervention dependent measures were the covariates for the post-intervention measures.
§Not significant (P > 0.05).

Table 3: Exercise Radionuclide Ventriculography

Index	Period	Experimental Group	Control Group	Significance*
Duration of exercise (seconds)	pre	392.1 ± 41.7	489.3 ± 39.3	P < 0.0001
	post	564.3 ± 54.0	483.9 ± 45.9	
Total work performed (kpm)	pre	2682.8 ± 392.7	3556.7 ± 500.3	P < 0.001
	post	4952.7 ± 542.4	3427.4 ± 443.5	
Maximum rate-pressure product (HR x BP x 10³) (beats/min x mm Hg)	pre	250.5 ± 10.2	223.5 ± 9.4	§NS
	post	251.0 ± 13.7	299.6 ± 12.9	

Data are presented as mean ± S.E.M.

*Changes in the experimental group were compared with changes in the control group using an analysis of covariance: the values of pre-intervention dependent measures were the covariates for the post-intervention measures.

§Not significant (P > 0.05)

Table 4: Medication Changes During the Intervention

	Discontinued	Reduced Dosage	No Change	Not Taking
Diuretics:				
Experimental	2	1	7	13
Control	0	0	5	18
Other antihypertensives:				
Experimental	2	1	7	13
Control	0	0	2	21
Beta-blockers:				
Experimental	4	8	3	8
Control	0	0	17	6

The control group remained essentially unchanged from 8.0 ± 2.1 episodes per week pre-intervention to 7.5 ± 2.1 post-intervention (F = 25.1, P < 0.0001).

Blood Pressure

It was necessary to discontinue antihypertensive medications and/or beta-blockers in 8 patients and reduce dosages in 10 others in the experimental group (Table 4) due to the appearance of medication side effects and/or hypotension (diastolic BP < 70 mm Hg), although none reported an increase in compliance to medication regimens during the intervention. No medication changes were made in control group patients. In the experimental group, propranolol was reduced in those taking it from a mean dosage of 80.7 mg per day to 40.7 mg per day; mean dosage in the control group remained unchanged (91.2 mg per day).

Despite these reductions in medications, the experimental group showed significant decreases in systolic (F = 1, P < 0.005) and diastolic (F = 9.3, P < 0.005) BP at rest and in response to various psychophysiological stimuli (Figure A-1), while the control group remained essentially unchanged (Figure A-2). The reduction in BP was greatest for those patients who were most hypertensive. In the eight patients who had a pre-intervention BP > 140 systolic or > 90 mm Hg diastolic, the resting BP was reduced from 156/97 to 120/80, and peak BP during the tasks was lowered from 182/116 to 153/94. In the control group, blood pressure did not change either at rest or during the tasks. There was a similar rise in stress-induced blood pressure in the experimental group in both the pre- and post-intervention studies (Figure A-1), but the post-intervention values were shifted downward on the ordinate, suggesting a possible reduction in general sympathetic tone.

Exercise Radionuclide Ventriculography

This test provides an accurate, non-invasive measure of left ventricular function at rest and during exercise. In interpreting the global left ventricular ejection fraction data, the *change* in ejection from rest to peak exercise (ΔEF) is more reflective of the degree of myocardial ischemia than the absolute values of ejection fraction at rest or at peak exercise. Most patients with multivessel IHD are unable to increase their ejection fraction more than 5 absolute percent from rest to peak exercise (ΔEF) and/or they exhibit new regional wall motion abnormalities during exercise that are not present at rest.[23–24]

Figure A-1. Blood Pressures: Responses to Psychological Stimuli Experimental Group

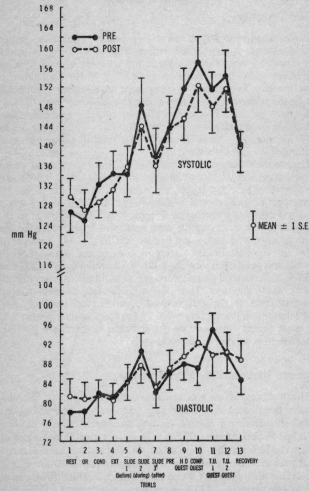

CONTROL GROUP

In Figures A-1 and A-2, the pre-intervention data are represented by solid lines and the post-intervention data by dotted lines. Results are expressed as mean ± S.E.M.

Appendix

Figure A-2. Blood Pressures: Responses to Psychological Stimuli
Control Group

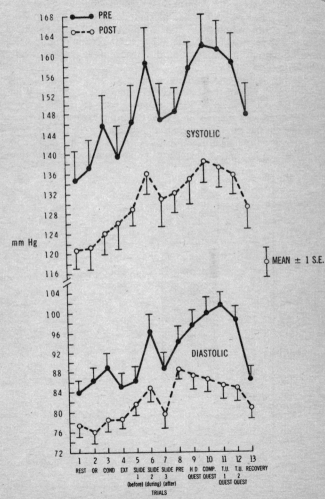

Appendix

EJECTION FRACTION RESPONSE

At pre-intervention, the ejection fraction response to exercise was abnormal for both the experimental and the control groups. In the experimental group, there was a slight decrease in mean ejection fraction from rest (58.8 ± 2.2 percent) to maximal exercise (57.9 ± 2.1 percent), $\Delta EF_{pre} = -0.6 \pm 1.5$ percent; in the control group there was a slight rise from rest (58.5 ± 1.7 percent) to maximal exercise (61.4 ± 2.2 percent), $\Delta EF_{pre} = +2.6 \pm 1.5$ percent (Figure A-3). These intergroup pre-intervention differences were not statistically significant (P > 0.05).

However, at post-intervention the mean ejection fraction response to exercise (ΔEF) of the experimental group was significantly improved when compared with the control group (F = 16.0, P < 0.0001, three-way analysis of variance). In the experimental group there was an increase in mean ejection fraction from rest (53.8 ± 2.4 percent) to maximal exercise (59.6 ± 2.7 percent) $\Delta EF_{post} = +5.8 \pm 1.5$ percent. In the control group there was less rise from

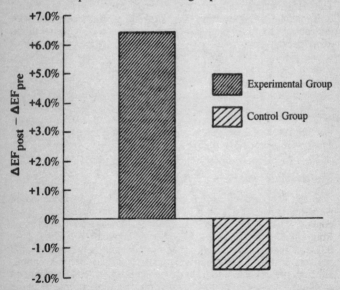

Figure A-3. Changes in Left Ventricular Ejection Fraction from Rest to Maximum Exercise (ΔEF) Pre/Post Intervention.

Each bar is obtained by subtracting ΔEF_{pre} from ΔEF_{post}, where ΔEF equals the change in ejection fraction from rest to peak exercise.

rest (56.3 ± 1.6 percent) to peak exercise (57.2 ± 2.4 percent) than in the pre-intervention studies, $\Delta EF_{post} = + 0.9$ percent.

In the experimental group, $\Delta EF_{post} - \Delta EF_{pre} = (+ 5.8)(-0.6) = + 6.4$ percent. Of these 23 patients, 19 showed improvement, 1 was unchanged, and 3 showed a slight decline (–1, –1, and –2 percent). In the control group, $\Delta EF_{post} - \Delta EF_{pre} = (+0.9)(+2.6) = -1.7$ percent. Of these 23 patients, 9 showed improvement, 1 was unchanged, and 13 showed decline (F = 12.5, P < 0.0001, analysis of covariance, Figure A-3).

Before the intervention, 20 patients in the experimental group and 15 patients in the control group demonstrated abnormal responses in the left ventricular ejection fraction to peak exercise ($\Delta EF < 5$ percent). After the intervention, only 10 patients in the experimental group exhibited abnormal ejection fraction responses to exercise, compared with 17 patients in the control group.

REGIONAL WALL MOTION

The experimental group also showed some improvements in regional wall motion at peak exercise post-intervention when compared with the control group. At pre-intervention, there were 13 patients in the experimental group with new regional wall motion abnormalities during peak exercise (not present at rest). Post-intervention, despite a much higher level of exercise, 5 of these displayed some improvement in regional wall motion when compared with their pre-intervention studies, 7 were unchanged, and 1 was worse (P < 0.05). At pre-intervention, 15 patients in the control group had new regional wall motion abnormalities during maximal exercise; post-intervention, 2 of these were somewhat improved, 6 were unchanged, and 7 were worse (P > 0.05).

Multivariate Analysis

In the experimental group, there was a significant reduction in weight during the intervention, from 172.8 ± 6.9 pounds to 162.5 ± 6.3 pounds, whereas the control group remained essentially unchanged from 181.5 ± 6.3 pounds to 183.0 ± 6.7 pounds (F = 79.3, P < 0.0001). Four of 9 smokers in the experimental group and 1 of 9 smokers in the control group quit smoking during the intervention, although they were not asked to do so. To assess whether weight and smoking reductions accounted for the observed improvements in the experimental group, we performed stepwise multiple regression analyses[33] individually with weight change and reduction in smoking as possible predictors of the observed changes (variance). Weight change as a predictor accounted for only 2 percent of the variance in ejection fraction changes, 9 percent of the variance in resting systolic, BP, 3 percent of the variance in total cholesterol, and none of the variance in total duration of exercise, total work performed, or diastolic BP. Smoking cessation as a predictor accounted for 8 percent of the variance in total cholesterol but was not a significant predictor for the variance in the other measured outcomes. Also, neither systolic nor diastolic BP changes were significant predictors of the variance in ejection fraction response, total duration of exercise, or total work performed.

DISCUSSION

Our study indicates that stress management training and a diet low in animal fat, cholesterol, and salt produced short-term improvements in patients with IHD when compared with a non-intervention control group. We measured statistically significant improvements in frequency of angina, total work performed, total duration of exercise, global left ventricular ejection fraction response to exercise, and regional wall motion response to exercise. The patients' cardiovascular risk status also improved as evidenced by reductions in plasma cholesterol, triglycerides, and both rest and reactivity measures of blood pressure when compared with the control group. Confidence in these findings is increased because patients were randomly assigned to group, medical tests were conducted by technicians blind to condition, and control patients did not improve. The data are consistent with our earlier pilot study.[35] The clinical significance of these changes remains to be determined. Regional wall motion and frequency of angina are subjectively assessed and are thus less rigorous than the other reported measures.

Many important questions remain unanswered. Our study was designed only to assess whether short-term improvements in cardiovascular function would result from these ancient and rather simple adjuncts to conventional treatments of IHD. It remains to be determined what the long-term effects would be. Also, our two-group design does not allow us to determine the relative contribution of each component of the intervention or the mechanisms of improvement. Further studies appear justified to explore these areas.

It is of particular interest from a cost-effective point of view to learn if the intervention can be equally effective and whether compliance can be maintained when taught on an outpatient basis rather than in a residential program. A recent report suggests that the effects of psychosocial environment in cardiovascular disease need to be considered. In this context, the group support, the close attention and encouragement given by the staff, and the pleasant environment may have contributed to the measured improvements.[36]

The improvements in global and regional left ventricular response to exercise occurred even though measured at much higher levels of exercise post-intervention. In patients with IHD, propranolol improves exercise tolerance and ventricular performance during exercise,[37] so it is of interest that the measured improvements occurred despite a substantial reduction in propranolol in many of the participants. Also, these changes were not correlated with reductions in blood pressure, weight, or smoking.

The possibility that changes in ejection fraction are due to factors other than an improvement in myocardial perfusion or performance should be considered. The ejection fraction change in the experimental group was due more to a reduction in resting ejection fraction post-intervention than to an increase in the ejection fraction at peak exercise. However, the control group also displayed a reduction in resting ejection fraction in the post-intervention studies (although somewhat less); when compared to this, the reduction in resting ejection fraction in the experimental group was not significant ($P > 0.05$). Other studies have demonstrated that the resting ejection fraction tends to be lower when it is measured a second time, whether by radionuclide ventriculography[38] or by coronary angiography.[39] This biologic variability may be related to greater familiarity with the procedures at the second study. Also, if the increase in the post-intervention ΔEF were due only to the decrease in resting ejection fraction, then the control group should have displayed a similar increase in the post-intervention ΔEF, but it did not. The changes are not likely due to a reduction in blood pressure (afterload), since neither systolic nor diastolic BP changes were significant predictors of the variance in ejection fraction response. Nevertheless, it is possible that the change in ejection fraction response may be due to factors other than a reduction in myocardial ischemia.

Aerobic exercise was not a component of this intervention, although some patients began to walk more as they became less symptom-limited. This may be responsible in part for the increase that we measured in total duration of exercise and total work performed. Although aerobic exercise has many cardiovascular benefits, it is not likely to be a factor in the short-term improvements in exercise radionuclide ventriculography that we measured.[40]

Our results are consistent with current concepts of the pathophysiology of IHD. There is some evidence to speculate that the apparent improvements in the experimental group may have occurred via currently accepted mechanisms of IHD, although we did not study this. Emotional stress may lead to myocardial ischemia both via coronary artery spasm and by increased platelet aggregation with coronary arteries.[41] Stress may lead to coronary spasm mediated either by direct alpha-adrenergic stimulation or secondary to the release of thromboxane A_2 from platelets, perhaps via increasing circulating catecholamines or other mediators.[42-48] Both thromboxane A_2 and catecholamines are potent constrictors of arterial smooth muscle and powerful endogenous stimulators of platelet aggregation.[49]

Even a single high-fat, high-cholesterol meal may cause acute enhancement of platelet reactivity.[50-52] These changes may result from a shift in the thromboxane/prostacyclin balance to favor thromboxane production; some evidence supports this. Cholesterol-enriched patelets release more arachidonic acid from platelet phospholipids than cholesterol-depleted platelets, and conversion of released arachidonic acid to platelet thromboxane is higher in cholesterol-rich platelets than in those that are cholesterol depleted.[53] In animals with atherosclerosis induced by high-cholesterol diets, platelets synthesize thromboxane A_2 in increased amounts.[54] Since cholesterol is contained only in foods of animal origin, a vegan diet may shift the balance away from thromboxane formation, which would make both coronary spasm and platelet aggregation less likely to occur.

In general, animal protein has been found to increase the level of plasma cholesterol, even in experiments in which the cholesterol and fat have been removed from the protein.[55] Some studies suggest that plant protein may be hypocholesterolemic.[56]

Changes in free fatty acid (FFA) metabolism may have contributed to the observed improvements. Myocardial oxygen is influenced by the substrate supply to the heart. Utilization of excess FFAs increases myocardial oxygen consumption and decreases left ventricular work, left ventricular systolic pressure, aortic pressure, epicardial motion, and exercise duration; these effects also are seen during myocardial ischemia.[57] Excess FFAs during ischemia result in even greater deteriorations in hemodynamic and metabolic functions.[58] A diet that contains a large proportion of animal products results in high blood levels of FFAs. The opposite is true with diets low in animal products, probably by shifting from noncarbohydrate to carbohydrate energy sources during physical or emotional stresses.[59] Emotional stress also increases blood levels of FFAs, primarily via catecholamine stimulation; further, catecholamines sensitize the heart to the oxygen-wasting effects of FFAs.[60]

In conclusion, a combination of stress management training and essentially vegan diet produced short-term improvement in cardiovascular status (as measured by a variety of endpoints) when compared to a non-intervention control group. Interpretation and generalization of these findings must be tempered with caution, since the patient population is selected and the sample size is relatively small. The intervention is safe and compatible with conventional treatments of IHD.

REFERENCES

1. Harvey W. Exercitatio de motu cordis et sanguinis. Cited in Eastwood MR, Trevelyan H. Stress and coronary heart disease. J. Psychosom Res. 1971; 15:289–92.

2. Osler W. The Lumleian lectures on angina pectoris. Lancet. 1910; 1:939.

3. Hackett TP, Rosenbaum JF. Emotion, psychiatric disorders, and the heart. In: Braunwald E, ed. Heart disease. Philadelphia: W.B. Saunders, 1980: 1923–43.

4. Orth-Gomer K, Ahlbom A. Impact of psychological stress on ischemic heart disease when controlling for conventional risk indicators. J Hum Stress. 1980; 6:7–15.

5. Eliot RS. Stress and the major cardiovascular disorders. Mount Kisco, New York: Futura Publishing, 1979.

6. Jenkins CD. Recent evidence supporting psychologic and social risk factors for coronary disease. N. Engl J. Med. 1976; 294:987–94, 1033–8.

7. Miller NE, Dworkin BR. Effects of learning on visceral functions—biofeedback. N Engl J. Med. 1977; 296:1274–8.

8. Benson H. Systemic hypertension and the relaxation response. N Engl J Med. 1977; 296: 1152–6.

9. Stone RA, DeLeo J. Psychotherapeutic control of hypertension. N Engl J Med. 1976; 294:80–4.

10. Patel CH, North WRS. Randomized controlled trial of yoga and biofeedback in the management of hypertension. Lancet. 1975; 2:93–5.

11. Shapiro AP, Schwartz GE, Ferguson DCE, Redmond DP, Weiss SM. Behavioral methods in the treatment of hypertension: a review of their clinical status. Ann Intern Med. 1977; 86:626–36.

12. Datey KK, Deshmukh SN, Dalvi CP, et al. Shavasan: a yogic exercise in the management of hypertension. Angiology. 1969; 20:325–33.

13. Patel CH. Reduction of serum cholesterol and blood pressure in hypertensive patients by behavior modification. J R Coll Gen Pract. 1976; 26:211–5.

Appendix

14. Cooper MJ, Aygen MM. A relaxation technique in the management of hypercholesterolemia. J Hum Stress. 1979; 4:24–7.

15. Keys A. Seven countries: a multivariate analysis of death and coronary heart disease. Cambridge: Harvard University Press, 1980: 212–35, 248–62, 315–43.

16. Gotto AM, Foreyt JP, Scott LW. Hyperlipidemia and nutrition: ongoing work. In: Hegyeli RJ, ed. Atherosclerosis Reviews. New York: Raven Press, 1980: 169–201.

17. Shekelle RB, Shyrock AM, Paul O, et al. Diet, serum cholesterol, and death from coronary heart disease: The Western Electric Study. N Engl J Med. 1981; 304:65–70.

18. Mahley RW. The role of dietary fat and cholesterol in atherosclerosis and lipoprotein metabolism. West J Med. 1981; 134:34–42.

19. Stamler J. Lifestyles, major risk factors, proof and public policy. Circulation. 1978; 58:3–19.

20. Sacks FM, Castelli WP, Donner A, Kass EH. Plasma lipids and lipoproteins in vegetarians and controls. N Engl J Med. 1975; 292:1148–51.

21. Sacks FM, Rosner B, Kass EH. Blood pressure in vegetarians, AM J Epidemiol. 1974; 100:390–8.

22. Ellis FR, Sanders T. Angina and vegan diet. Am Heart J. 1977; 93:803–5.

23. Okada RD, Boucher CA, Strauss HW, Pohost GM. Exercise radionuclide imaging approaches to coronary artery disease. Amer J Cardiol. 1980; 46:1188–1204.

24. Borer JS, Bacharach SL, Green MV, et al. Real-time radionuclide cineangiography in the noninvasive evaluation of global and regional left ventricular function at rest and during exercise in patients with coronary-artery disease. N Engl J Med. 1977; 296:839–44.

25. Fuhrer MJ, Baer PE, Cowan CO. Orienting responses and personality variables as predictors of differential conditioning of electrodermal responses and awareness of stimulus reactions. J Pers and Soc Psychol. 1973; 27:287–96.

26. Rosenman RH. The interview method of assessment of the coronary-prone behavior pattern. In: Dembroski TM, Weiss SM, Shields JL, Haynes SG, Fienleib M, eds. Coronary prone behavior. New York: Springer-Verlag, 1978:55–69.

27. Manual of laboratory operations, Lipid Research Clinics Program. Vol. 1 Lipid and lipoprotein analysis. Washington, D.C.: Government Printing Office, DHEW publication No. (NIH) 75–628, 1974.

Appendix

28. Ornish D. Mind/heart interactions: for better and for worse. Health Values. 1978; 2:266–9.
29. Satchidananda S. Integral yoga hatha. New York: Holt, Rinehart and Winston, 1970:11–25, 41–52, 54, 62, 82, 84–5.
30. Carrington P. Freedom in meditation. New York: Anchor Press/Doubleday, 1977.
31. Easwaren E. Meditation. Petaluma, California: Nilgiri Press, 1978.
32. Samuels M, Samuels N. Seeing with the mind's eye. New York: Random House, 1975: 208–38.
33. Nie NH. SPSS: Statistical package for the social sciences, 2nd ed. New York: McGraw-Hill, 1975:320–67, 398–433.
34. Dixon WJ, ed. Biomedical computer programs. Berkeley: Univ of Calif Press, 1975:711.
35. Ornish DM, Gotto AM, Miller RR, Rochelle D, McAllister GK. Effects of a vegetarian diet and selected yoga techniques in the treatment of coronary heart disease. Clinical Research. 1979; 27:720A.
36. Nerem RM, Levesque MJ, Cornhill JF. Social environment as a factor in diet-induced atherosclerosis. Science. 1980; 208:1475–6.
37. Marshall RC, Wisenberg G, Schelbert R, Henze E. Effect of oral propanolol on rest, exercise and post-exercise left ventricular performance in normal subjects and patients with coronary artery disease. Circulation. 1981; 63:572–83.
38. Upton MT, Rerych SK, Newman GE, Bounous EP, Jones RH. The reproductibility of radionuclide angiographic measurements of left ventricular function in normal subjects at rest and during exercise. Circulation. 1981; 62:126–32.
39. McAnulty JH, Kremkau EL, Rosch J. Hattenhauer MT, Rahimtoola SH. Spontaneous changes in left ventricular function between sequential studies. Amer J Cardiol. 1974; 34:23–8.
40. Verani MS, Hartung GH, Harris JK, Welton DE, Pratt CM, Miller RR. Effects of exercise training on left ventricular performance and myocardial perfusion in patients with coronary artery disease. Amer J Cardiol. 1981; 47:797–803.
41. Oliva PB. Pathophysiology of acute infarction, 1981. Ann Intern Med. 1981; 94:236–250.
42. Hirsh PD, Hillis LD, Campbell WB, Firth BG, Willerson JT. Release of prostaglandins and thromboxane into the coronary circulation in patients with ischemic heart disease. N Engl J Med. 1981; 304:685–91.
43. Schiffer F, Hartley LH, Schulman CL, Abelmann WH. Evidence for emotionally-induced coronary arterial spasm in patients with angina pectoris. Br Heart J. 1980; 44:62–6.

Appendix

44. Haft JI, Arkel YS. Effect of emotional stress on platelet aggregation in humans. Chest. 1976; 70:501–5.

45. Arkel YS, Haft JI, Kreutner W, Sherwood J, Williams R. Alteration in second phase platelet aggregation associated with an emotionally stressful activity. Thromb Haemostas. 1977; 38:552–61.

46. Haft JI, Fani K. Intravascular platelet aggregation in the heart induced by stress. Circulation. 1973; 47:353–8.

47. Warltier DC, Zyvoloski M, Garrett JG, Hardman HF, Brooks HL. Redistribution of myocardial blood flow distal to a dynamic coronary aterial stenosis by sympathomimetic amines. Amer J Cardiol. 1981; 48:269–79.

48. Williams DO, Most AS. Responsiveness of the coronary circulation to brief vs sustained alpha-adrenergetic stimulation. Circulation. 1980; 63:11–16.

49. Moncada S, Vane JR. Arachidonic acid metabolites and the interactions between platelets and blood vessel walls. N Engl J Med. 1979; 300:1142–7.

50. Haft JI. Role of blood platelets in coronary artery disease. Amer J Cardiol. 1979; 43:1197–1206.

51. Horlick L. Platelet adhesiveness in normal persons and subjects with atherosclerosis: effects of high fat meals and anticoagulants on the adhesive index. Amer J Cardiol. 1961; 8: 459–70.

52. Moolton SE, Jennings PB, Solden A. Dietary fat and platelet adhesiveness in ateriosclerosis and diabetes. Amer J Cardiol. 1963; 11:290–300.

53. Stuart JM, Gerrard JM, White JG. Effects of cholesterol on production of thromboxane B_2 by platelets in vitro. N Engl J Med. 1980; 302:6–10.

54. Zmuda A, Dembinska-Kiec A, Chytkowski A, Gryglewski RJ. Experimental atherosclerosis in rabbits. Prostaglandins. 1977; 14:1035–43.

55. Carroll KK. Dietary protein in relation to plasma cholesterol levels and atherosclerosis. Nutr Reviews. 1978; 36:1–5.

56. Sirtori CR, Agradi E, Conti F, Mantero O, Gatti E. Soybean-protein diet in the treatment of type-II hyper lipoproteinemia. Lancet. 1977; 1:275–7.

57. Simonsen S, Kjekshus JK. The effect of free fatty acids on myocardial oyxgen consumption during atrial pacing and catecholamine infusion in man. Circulation. 1978; 58:484–91.

58. Liedtke AJ, Nellis S, Neely JR. Effects of free fatty acids on mechanical and metabolic function in normal and ischemic myocardium in swine. Circ Res. 1978; 43:652–61.

Appendix

59. Martin B, Robinson S, Robertshaw D. Influence of diet on leg uptake of glucose during heavy exercise. Am J Clin Nutr. 1978; 31:62–7.

60. Vik-Mo H, Mjos OD. Influence of free fatty acids on myocardial oxygen consumption and ischemic injury. Amer J Cardiol. 1981; 48:361–5.

Selected Bibliography

INTRODUCTION

Ellis FR, Sanders T. Angina and vegan diet. American Heart Journal. 1977; 93:803–5.

Kritchevsky D. Soya, saponins, and plasma cholesterol. Lancet. 1979; i:610.

Sacks FM, Castelli WP, Donner A, Kass EH. Plasma lipids on lipoproteins in vegetarians and controls. New England Journal of Medicine. 1975; 292:1148–51.

Sacks, FM, Rosner B, Kass EH. Blood pressure in vegetarians. American Journal of Epidemiology. 1974; 100:390–8.

Sacks FM, Donner A, Castelli WP, et al. Effect of ingestion of meat on plasma cholesterol of vegetarians. JAMA. 1981; 246:604–4.

1. OVERVIEW

Blacher RS, Cleveland RJ. Heart surgery. JAMA. 1979; 242:2463–4.

Blacher RS. The hidden psychosis of open-heart surgery, with a note on the sense of awe. JAMA. 1972; 222:305–6.

Block TA, Murray JA, English MT. Improvement in exercise performance after unsuccessful myocardial revascularization. American Jouranl of Cardiology. 1977; 40:673.

Bourassa MG, Lesperance J, Corbara F, et al. Progression of obstructive coronary artery disease 5 to 7 years after aortocoronary bypass surgery. Circulation (supp.1). 1978; 58:100–106.

Braunwald E, ed. Heart disease. Philadelphia: W.B. Saunders Co., 1980.

Selected Bibliography

Cobb LA. An evaluation of internal-mammary artery ligation by a double blind technique. New England Journal of Medicine. 1959; 260:1115–8.

Diet and cancer: what do we know so far? Your Patient and Cancer. 1982; 2:49–59.

Hjermann I, Velve Byre K, Holme I, Leren P. Effect on diet and smoking intervention on the incidence of coronary heart disease. Lancet. 1981; ii:1303–10.

Kramer JR, Matsuda Y, Mulligan JC, et al. Progression for coronary atherosclerosis. Circulation. 1981; 63:519.

Lawrie GM, Morris GC, Howell JF, et al. Results of coronary bypass more than 5 years after operation in 434 patients. American Journal of Cardiology. 1977; 40:665.

Lown B, Verrier RL, Rabinowitz SH. Neural and psychological mechanisms and the problem of sudden cardiac death. American Journal of Cardiology. 1977; 39:890–902.

McIntosh HD, Garcia JA. The first decade of aortocoronary bypass grafting, 1967–1977: a review. Circulation. 1978; 57:405–31.

Medical News. Regression of atherosclerosis: preliminary but encouraging news. JAMA. 1981; 246:2309–12.

Moore RB, Buchwald H, Varco RL. The effect of partial ileal bypass on plasma lipoproteins. Circulation. 1980; 62:469.

National Academy of Sciences. Diet, nutrition, and cancer. Washington: National Academy Press, 1982.

National Academy of Sciences. Health and behavior. Washington: National Academy Press, 1982.

Ornish DM, Scherwitz L, Doody R, Kesten D, McLanahan S, Brown S, DePuey EG, Sonnemaker R, Haynes C, Lester J, Dutton L, McAllister G, Baer P, Hall RD, Burdine J, Gotto AM. Effects of stress management techniques and dietary changes in treating ischemic heart disease. American Journal of Cardiology. 1982; 49:1008.

Ornish DM, Gotto AM, Miller RR, Rochelle D, McAllister GK. Effects of a vegetarian diet and selected yoga techniques in the treatment of coronary heart disease. Clinical Research. 1979; 27:720A.

Pasternak R, Cohn K, Selzer A, Langston MF. Enhanced rate of progression of coronary artery disease following aortocoronary saphenous vein bypass surgery. American Journal of Cardiology. 1975; 58:166–170.

Roth D, Kostuk WJ. Noninvasive and invasive demonstration of spontaneous regression of coronary artery disease. Circulation. 1980; 62:888–96.

Selected Bibliography

Stamler J. Lifestyles, major risk factors, proof and public policy. Circulation. 1978; 58:3–19.

U.S. Department of Health and Human Services Monthly Vital Statistics Report: Final Mortality Statistics. Hyattsville, Maryland: National Center of Health Statistics, 1978.

3. OBJECTIVE IMPROVEMENTS

Bodenheimer MM, Banka VS, Fooshee CM, Helfant RH. Comparative sensitivity of the exercise electrocardiogram, thallium imaging and stress radionuclide angiography to detect the presence and severity of coronary heart disease. Circulation. 1979; 60:1270.

Borer JS, Bacharach SL, Green MV, et al. Real-time radionuclide cineangiography in the noninvasive evaluation of global and regional left ventricular function at rest and during exercise in patients with coronary-artery disease. New England Journal of Medicine. 1977; 296:839–44.

Hartley LH. Prescribing physical conditioning activity. Practical Cardiology. 1981; 7:119–129.

Kramsch DM, Aspen AJ, Abramowitz BM, et al. Reduction of coronary atherosclerosis by moderate conditioning exercise in monkeys on an atherogenic diet. New England Journal of Medicine. 1981; 305:1483–9.

Paffenbarger RS, Hale WE. Work activity and coronary heart mortality. New England Journal of Medicine. 1975; 292:545.

Paffenbarger RS, Wing AL, Hyde RT. Physical activity as an index of heart attack risk in college alumni. American Journal of Epidemiology. 1978; 108:161–175.

Thomas GS, Lee PR, Franks P, Paffenberger RS. Exercise and health: the evidence and the implications. Cambridge: Oelgeschlager, Gunn & Hain, Inc., 1981.

Verani MS, Hartung GH, Harris JK, Welton DE, Pratt CM, Miller RR. Effects of exercise training on left ventricular performance and myocardial perfusion in patients with coronary artery disease. American Journal of Cardiology. 1981; 47:797–803.

4. WHAT IS CORONARY HEART DISEASE AND HOW DO STRESS AND DIET HELP TO CAUSE IT?

Also see references at end of the appendix.

Adsett CA. Changes in coronary blood flow and other demodynamic indicators induced by stressful interviews. Psychosomatic Medicine. 1962; 24:331–336.

Selected Bibliography

American Dietetic Association. Position paper on the vegetarian approach to eating. J Am Dietet A. 1980; 77:61–69.

Ardlie NG, Glew G, Schwartz CJ. Influence of catecholamines on nucleotide-induced platelet aggregation. Nature. 1966; 212:415–17.

Arkel YS, Haft J, Kreutner W, Sherwood J, Williams R. Alteration in second phase platelet aggregation associated with an emotionally stressful activity. Thrombosis and Hemostasis. 1977; 38:552.

Axelrod PJ, Verrier RL, Lown B. Vulnerability to ventricular fibrillation during acute coronary occlusion and release. American Journal of Cardiology. 1975; 36:776.

Barndt R, Blankenhorn DH, Crawford DW, Brooks SH. Regression and progression of early femoral atherosclerosis in treated hyperlipoproteinemic patients. Annals of Internal Medicine. 1977; 86:139–46.

Bassan MM, Marcus HS, Ganz W. The effect of mild-to-moderate mental stress on coronary hemodynamics in patients with coronary artery disease. Circulation. 1980; 65:933–5.

Basset JR, Caincross KD. Changes in the coronary vascular system following prolonged exposure to stress. Pharmacol. Biochem. Behav. 1977; 6:311.

Blankenhorn DH, Brooks SH. Angiographic trials of lipid-lowering therapy. Arteriosclerosis. 1981; 1:242–9.

Brody J. Researcher traces a process of cholesterol buildup. New York Times, June 18, 1981, p. A27.

Bruhn JG, Paredes A, Adsett CA, Wolf S. Psychological predictors of sudden death in myocardial infarction. J. Psychosom. Res. 1974; 18:187–91.

Burslem J, Schonfeld G, Howald MA, Weidman SW, Miller JP. Plasma apoprotein and lipoprotein lipid levels in vegetarians. Metabolism. 1978; 27:711.

Cannon WB. The emergency function of the adrenal medulla in pain and the major emotions. American Journal of Physiology. 1914; 33:356–372.

Cannon WB. Bodily changes in pain, hunger, fear, and rage. New York: Appleton, 1929.

Carey RJ. Self-predicted fatal myocardial infarction in absence of coronary artery disease. Lancet. 1980; i:January 19, 1980, p. 159.

Carroll KK. Dietary protein in relation to plasma cholesterol levels and artherosclerosis. Nutrition Reviews. 1978; 36:1–5.

DeBakey ME, Gotto AM. The living heart. New York: Grosset and Dunlap, 1977.

DeSilva RA, Lown B. Ventricular premature beats, stress, and sudden death. Psychosomatics. 1978; 19:649–61.

Selected Bibliography

Dimsdale JE. Emotional causes of sudden death. American Journal of Psychiatry. 1977; 134:12.

Eliot RS. What I learned from my MI. Modern Medicine. 1981; 49:62–72.

El-Maraghi NR, Sealey BJ. Recurrent myocardial infarction in a young man due to coronary arterial spasm demonstrated at autopsy. Circulation. 1980; 61:199.

Engel GL. Sudden and rapid death during psychological stress: folklore or folk wisdom? Annals of Internal Medicine. 1971; 74:771–82.

Engel GL. Psychologic factors in instantaneous cardiac death. New England Journal of Medicine. 1976; 294:664–5.

Fozzard HA. Electrophysiology of the heart: the effects of ischemia. Hospital Practice. May 1980; pp. 61–71.

Friedman M, Byers SO, Brown AE. Plasma lipid responses of rats and rabbits to an auditory stimulus. American Journal of Physiology. 1967; 212:1174.

Fuller CM, Raizner AE, Chahine RA, et al. Exercise-induced coronary arterial spasm. American Journal of Cardiology. 1980; 46:500.

Fuster V, Chesebro JH, Frye RL, Elveback LR. Platelet survival and the development of coronary artery disease in the young adult. Circulation. 1981; 63:546.

Garfield CA. Stress and survival: the emotional realities of life-threatening illness. St. Louis: C.V. Mosby, 1979.

Gertz SD, Uretsky G, Wajnberg RS, Navot N, Gotsman MS. Endothelial cell damage and thrombus formation after partial arterial constriction: relevance to the role of coronary artery spasm in the pathogenesis of myocardial infarction. Circulation. 1981; 63:476.

Goldstein S. Sudden death and coronary heart disease. Mt. Kisco, New York: Futura, 1974.

Gotto AM. Regression of atherosclerosis. American Journal of Medicine. 1981; 70:989–991.

Graboys TB. Celtics fever: playoff-induced ventricular arrhythmia. New England Journal of Medicine. 1981; 305:467–8.

Green LH, Seroppian E, Handin RI. Platelet activation during exercise-induced myocardial ischemia. New England Journal of Medicine. 1980; 302:193–7.

Haft JI, Fani K. Intravascular platelet aggregation in the heart induced by stress. Circulation. 1973; 47:353–8.

Haft, JI, Fani K. Stress and the induction of intravascular platelet aggregation in the heart. Circulation. 1973; 48:164–8.

Selected Bibliography

Haft JI, Arkel YS. Effect of emotional stress on platelet aggregation in humans. Chest. 1976; 70:501.

Haft JI. Role of blood patelets in coronary artery disease. American Journal of Cardiology. 1979; 43:1197–1205.

Harlan WR. Physical and psychosocial stress and the cardiovascular system. Circulation. 1981; 63:266A.

Havlik RJ, Feinleib M. Proceedings of the conference on the decline in coronary heart disease mortality. Washington: NIH publication #79-1610, 1979.

Hegyeli RJ. Atherosclerosis reviews, volume 7. New York: Raven Press, 1980.

Helfant RH. Coronary spasm. American Journal of Cardiology. 1979; 44:839–41.

Hellstrom HR. Coronary artery vasospasm: the likely immediate cause of acute myocardial infarction. British Heart Journal. 1979; 41:426–32.

Heupler FA. Syndrome of symptomatic coronary artery spasm with nearly normal coronary arteriograms. American Journal of Cardiology. 1980; 45:873.

Horlick L. Platelet adhesiveness in normal persons and subjects with atherosclerosis. Effect of high fat meals and anticoagulants on the adhesive index. American Journal of Cardiology. 1961; 18:459.

Hurley R. American Heart Association heartbook. New York: E.P. Dutton, 1980.

Jarvinen KAJ. Can ward rounds be a danger to patients with myocardial infarction? British Medical Journal. 1955; 1:318–20.

Johnson RA, Haber E, Austen WG. The practice of cardiology. Boston: Little, Brown and Company, 1980.

Kannel WB. Prospects for risk factor modification to reduce risk of reinfarction and premature death. Journal of Cardiac Rehabilitation. 1981; 1:63.

Kumpuris AG, Luchi RJ, Waddell CC, Miller RR. Production of circulating platelet aggregates by exercise in coronary patients. Circulation. 1980; 61:162.

Levy RI, Rifkin BM, Dennis BH, Ernst ND. Nutrition, lipids, and coronary heart disease: a global view. New York: Raven Press, 1979.

Liang B, Verrier RL, Melman J, Lown B. Correlation between circulating catecholamine levels and ventircular vulnerability during psychological stress in conscious dogs. Proceedings for the Society for Experimental Biology and Medicine. 1979; 161:266–9.

Selected Bibliography

Lown B, Temte JV, Reich P, Gaughan C, Regenstein Q, Hai H. Basis for recurring ventricular fibrillation in the absence of coronary heart disease and its management. New England Journal of Medicine. 1976; 294:623–9.

Lown B, Verrier R. Neural activity and ventricular fibrillation. New England Journal of Medicine. 1976; 294:1165–70.

Lown B. Sudden cardiac death: the major challenge confronting contemporary cardiology. American Journal of Cardiology. 1979; 43:313.

Lown B. Sudden cardiac death—1978. Circulation. 1979; 60:1593–99.

Lown B, DeSilva RA, Reich P, Murawski BJ. Psychophysiologic factors in sudden cardiac death. American Journal of Psychiatry. 1980; 137:1325–35.

Lown B. The role of the autonomic nervous system in the pathogenesis of arrhythmias. American College of Cardiology annual convention, Houston, Texas, March 10, 1980.

Lown B, DeSilva RA. Is coronary arterial spasm a risk factor for coronary atherosclerosis? American Journal of Cardiology. 1980; 45:901.

Luchi RJ, Chahine RA. Coronary artery spasm. Annals of Internal Medicine. 1979; 91:441–449.

Lynch JJ, Thomas SA, Paskewitz DA, Katcher AH, Weir LO. Human contact and cardiac arrhythmia in a coronary care unit. Psychosomatic Medicine. 1977; 39:188–192.

Mahley RW. The role of dietary fat and cholesterol in atherosclerosis and lipoprotein metabolism. Western Journal of Medicine. 1981; 139:34.

Marmot MG, Syme SL, Kagan A, Kato H, Cohen JB, Belsky J. Epidemiologic studies of coronary heart disease and stroke in Japanese men living in Japan, Hawaii, and California. American Journal of Epidemiology. 1975; 102:514–25.

Martin B, Robinson S, Robertshaw D. Influence of diet on leg uptake of glucose during heavy exercise. American Journal of Clinical Nutrition. 1978; 31:62–7.

Marx JL. Coronary artery spasm and heart disease. Science. 1980; 208:1127–30.

Marzilli M, Goldstein S, Trivella M, Palumbo C, Maseri A. Some clinical considerations regarding the relation of coronary vasospasm to coronary atherosclerosis: a hypothetical pathogenesis. American Journal of Cardiology. 1980; 45:882–903.

Maseri A, L'Abbate A, Baroldi G, et al. Coronary vasospasm as a possible cause of myocardial infarction. New England Journal of Medicine. 1978; 299:1271–7.

Selected Bibliography

Mehta J, Mehta P. Role of blood platelets and prostaglandins in coronary artery disease. American Journal of Cardiology. 1981; 48:366.

Moolten SE, Jennings PB, Solden A. Dietary fat and platelet adhesiveness in arteriosclerosis and diabetes. American Journal of Cardiology. 1969 11:290–303.

Morgan T, Myers J, Carney S. The evidence that salt is an important etiological agent, if not the cause, of hypertension. Clinical Science. 1979; 57:459s–462.

Moss A, Wynar B. Tachycardia in house officers presenting cases at Grand Rounds. Annals of Internal Medicine. 1970; 72:255–6.

Oliva PB. Pathophysiology of acute myocardial infarction, 1981. Annals of Internal Medicine. 1981; 94:236–250.

Oliva PB, Breckinridge JC. Acute myocardial infarction with normal and near normal coronary arteries. American Journal of Cardiology. 1977; 40:1000.

Orme-Johnson DW, Farrow JT. Scientific research on the TM program, vol. 1. Livingston Manor, N.Y.: Maharishi University Press, 1977.

Parfrey PS, Wright P, Goodwin FJ, et al. Blood pressure and hormonal changes following alteration in dietary sodium and potassium in mild essential hypertension. Lancet, 1981; i:59–63.

Patel CH. Reduction of serum cholesterol and blood pressure in hypertensive patients by behavior modification. Journal of the Royal College of General Practitioners. 1976; 26:211–15.

Rahe RH, Romo M, Bennett L, et al. Recent life changes, myocardial infarction and abrupt coronary death. Archives of Internal Medicine. 1974; 133:221–8.

Reich P, DeSilva RA, Lown B, Murawski BJ. Acute psychological disturbances preceding life-threatening ventricular arrhythmias. JAMA. 1981; 233–5.

Ross R, Harker L. Hyperlipidemia and atherosclerosis. Science. 1976; 193:1094–1100.

Ross R, Glomset JA. The pathogenesis of atherosclerosis. New England Journal of Medicine, 1976; 295:369–77, 420–5.

Satinsky J, Kowsowsky B, Lown B. Ventricular fibrillation induced by hypothalamic stimulation during coronary occlusion. Circulation, Supplement II. 1971, p.II–60.

Schiffer F, Hartley LH, Schulman CL, Abelmann WH. Evidence for emotionally-induced coronary arterial spasm in patients with angina pectoris. British Heart Journal. 1980; 44:62–6.

Scott NA, DeSilva RA, Lown B, Wurtman RJ. Tyrosine administration decreases vulnerability to ventricular fibrillation in the normal canine heart. Science. 1981; 211;727–9.

Selected Bibliography

Selye H. Selye's guide to stress research, vol. 1. New York: Van Nostrand Reinhold Co., 1980.

Simonsen S, Kjekshus JK. The effect of free fatty acids on myocardial oxygen consumption during atrial pacing and catecholamine infusion in man. Circulation. 1978; 58:484.

Sirtori CR, Agradi E, Conti F, Mantero O, Gatti E. Soybean-protein diet in the treatment of type II hyperlipoproteinemia. Lancet. 1977; i:275–7.

Sirtori CR, Gatti MD, Mantero O, et al. Clinical experience with the soybean protein diet in the treatment of hypercholesterolemia. American Journal of Clinical Nutrition. 1979; 32:1645–1658.

Skinner JE, Lie JT, Entman ML. Modification of ventricular fibrillation latency following coronary artery occlusion in the conscious pig. Circulation. 1975; 51:656–67.

Skinner JE, Reed JC. Blockage of frontocortical-brainstem pathway prevents ventricular fibrillation of ischemic heart. American Journal of Physiology. 1981; 240:H156–63.

Small DM. Cellular mechanisms for lipid deposition in atherosclerosis. New England Journal of Medicine. 1977; 297:873.

Steele P, Rainwater J. Effects of dietary and pharmacologic alteration of serum lipids on platelet survival time. Circulation. 1978; 58:365.

Steinberg D. Research related to underlying mechanisms in atherosclerosis. Circulation. 1979; 60:1559.

Stuart MJ, Gerrard JM, White JG. Effect of cholesterol on production of thromboxane B_2 by platelets in vitro. New England Journal of Medicine. 1980; 302:6–10.

Taggart P, Carruthers M, et al. Electrocardiographic changes resembling myocardial ischemia in asymptomatic men with normal coronary arteriograms. British Heart Journal. 1979; 41:214–25.

Turpeinen O. Effect of cholesterol-lowering diet on mortality from coronary heart disease and other causes. Circulation. 1979; 59:1–7.

Vik-Mo H, Mjos OD. Influence of free fatty acids on myocardial oxygen consumption and ischemic injury. American Journal of Cardiology. 1981; 48:361.

Warltier DC, Zyvoloski M, Gross GJ, et al. Redistribution of myocardial blood flow distal to a dynamic coronary arterial stenosis by sympathomimetic amines. American Journal of Cardiology. 1981; 48:269.

Weiner L, Kasparian H, Duca PR, et al. Spectrum of coronary arterial spasm. American Journal of Cardiology. 1976; 38:945.

Wissler RW, Vesselinovitch D. Regression of atherosclerosis in experimental animals and man. Modern Concepts of Cardiovascular Disease. 1977; 46:27.

Wolf S. The end of the rope: the role of the brain in cardiac death. Canadian Medical Association Journal, 1967; 97:1022.

Wurtmann R. Use of nutrients to modify neurotransmission. Medical Grand Rounds, Massachusetts General Hospital, December 24, 1981.

5. ASSUMPTIONS: WHY DO WE FEEL STRESS?

Adler J. Stress: how it can hurt. Newsweek magazine. April 21, 1980, pp. 106–8.

DeVries M. The redemption of the intangible in medicine. London: The Institute of Psychosynthesis, 1981.

Dostoyevsky F. Notes from underground. New York: New American Library, 1961.

Easwaran E. Dialogue with death. Petaluma, California: Nilgiri Press, 1981.

Ferguson M. The Aquarian conspiracy. Los Angeles: J.P. Tarcher, Inc., 1980.

Friedman E, Katcher AH, Lynch JJ, Thomas SA. Animal companions and one-year survival of patients after discharge from a coronary care unit. Public Health Reports, 1980; 95:307.

Friedman M. Rosenman RH. Type A behavior and your heart. New York: Alfred A. Knopf, 1974.

Isherwood C. How to know God. New York: New American Library, 1953.

Kuhn TS. The structure of scientific revolutions. Chicago: University of Chicago Press, 1962.

Lynch JJ. The broken heart: the medical consequences of loneliness. New York: Basic Books, Inc., 1977.

Mandelkorn P. To know your self. Garden City, New York: Anchor Press, 1978.

Nerem RM, Levesque MJ, Cornhill JF. Social environment as a factor in diet-induced atherosclerosis. Science. 1980; 208:1475–6.

Ornish D. Mind/heart interactions: for better and for worse. Health Values. 1978; 2:266–9.

Powell L. Indicators of the Type A behavior pattern and the incidence of recurring coronary heart disease. Dissertation, Stanford University, 1981.

Reed JD. America shapes up. Time magazine. November 2, 1981, pp. 94–106.

Remen N. The human patient. New York: Anchor Press/Doubleday, 1980.

Selected Bibliography

Rose RM, Jenkins CD, Hurst MW. Health change in air traffic controllers: a prospective study. Psychosomatic Medicine. 1978; 40:142–65.

Scherwitz L, Berton K, Leventhal H. Type A behavior, self-involvement, and cardiovascular response. Psychosomatic Medicine. 1978; 40:593–609.

Scherwitz L, McKelvain R, Laman C, et al. Type A behavior, self-involvement, and coronary atherosclerosis. Psychosomatic Medicine. 1983; in press.

Vaillant GE. Natural history of male psychologic health: effects of mental health on physical health. New England Journal of Medicine. 1979; 301:1249–54.

Vivekananda S. Jnana yoga. New York: Ramakrishna-Vivekananda Center, 1970.

Wolf S, Goodell H. Behavioral science in clinical medicine. Springfield, Illinois: Charles Thomas, Inc., 1976, pp. 17–18.

PART II. STRESS MANAGEMENT TECHNIQUES

Achterberg J, Lawlis GF. Bridges of the bodymind. Champaign, Illinois: Institute for Personality and Ability Testing, Inc., 1980.

Albrink MJ, Newman T, Davidson PC. Effect of high and low-fiber diets on plasma lipids and insulin. American Journal of Clinical Nutrition. 1979; 32:1486.

Anderson B. Stretching. New York: Random House, 1980.

Ballentine R. Diet and nutrition. Honesdale, Pennsylvania: Himalayan International Institute, 1978.

Bargen R. The vegetarian's self-defense manual. Wheaton, Illinois: Quest Books, 1979.

Benson H. The relaxation response. New York: William Morrow and Co., 1975.

Benson H. Systemic hypertension and the relaxation response. New England Journal of Medicine. 1977; 296:1152–6.

Benson H. The mind/body effect. New York: Simon and Schuster, 1979.

Benson H, Alexander S, Feldman CL. Decreased premature ventricular contractions through the use of the relaxation response in patients with stable ischemic heart disease. Lancet. 1979; ii:380.

Benson H, Rosner BA, Marzetta BR, et al. Decreased blood pressure in borderline hypertensive subjects who practiced meditation. J. Chronic Dis. 1974; 27:163–9.

Berry R. The vegetarians. Brookline: Autumn Press, 1979.

Selected Bibliography

Bhajan Y. The Golden Temple vegetarian cookbook. New York: Hawthorn Books, 1978.

Bohls K. Using visualization, Utah State QB sets sights on UT win. Austin: Austin American Statesman, September 20, 1980, p. D3.

Brena S. Yoga and medicine. New York: Julian Press, 1970.

Bricklin M, Claessens S. The natural healing cookbook. Emmaus, Pennsylvania: Rodale Press, 1981.

Brody J. Jane Brody's nutrition book. New York: W.W. Norton and Company, 1981.

Brown EE. The Tassajara bread book. Berkeley: Shambhala Publications, Inc., 1970 (distributed by Random House).

Bry A. Directing the movies of your mind. Scranton, Pennsylvania: Harper and Row, 1978.

Burrow J, Norwak M. Health food cookbook. London: Octopus Books, 1979.

Carrington P, Collings GH, Benson H, et al. The use of meditation/relaxation techniques for the management of stress in a working population. Journal of Occupational Medicine. 1980; 22:221.

Christensen A, Rankin D. Easy does it yoga. San Francisco: Harper and Row, 1975.

Cooper MJ, Aygen MM. A relaxation technique in the management of hyper-cholesterolemia. J. Hum Stress. 1979; 4:24–7.

Cousins N. Anatomy of an illness as perceived by the patient. New York: W.W. Norton, 1979.

Datey KK, Deshmukh SN, Dalvi CP, et al. Shavasan: a yogic exercise in the management of hypertension. Angiology. 1969; 20:325–33.

Dawber TR. The Framingham study. Cambridge: Harvard University Press, 1980.

Doyle R. The vegetarian handbook. New York: Crown Publishers, 1979.

Eckardt MJ, Harford TC, Kaelber Ct, et al. Health hazards associated with alcohol consumption. JAMA. 1981; 246:648–666.

Eliot RS. Stress and the major cardiovascular disorders. Mt. Kisco, New York: Futura Publishing, 1979.

Ford MW, Hillyard S, Kooch MF. Deaf Smith county cookbook. New York: Macmillan, 1973.

Funderburk J. Science studies yoga; a review of physiological data. Honesdale, Pennsylvania: Himalayan International Institute, 1977.

Gordon T, Kagan A, Garcia-Palmieri M. Diet and its relation to coronary heart disease and death in three populations. Circulation. 1981; 63:500.

Selected Bibliography

Gravenstein JS, Kalhan S, Balamoutsos NG. Of breath and spirits. JAMA. 1981; 246:1091–2.

Greenspon AJ, Stang JM, Lewis RP, Schaal SF. Provocation of ventricular tachycardia after consumption of alcohol. New England Journal of Medicine. 1979; 301:1049.

Haggerty RJ. Life stress, illness, and social supports. Develop. Med. Child Neurol. 1980; 22:391–400.

Hartbarger JC, Hartbarger NJ. Eating for the eighties. Philadelphia: W.B. Saunders Company, 1981.

Jacob RG, Kraemer HC, Agras WS. Relaxation therapy in the treatment of hypertension—a review. Archives of General Psychiatry. 1977; 34:1417–27.

Jacobsen E. Progressive relaxation. Chicago: University of Chicago Press, 1938.

Jacobsen E. You must relax (5th ed). New York: McGraw-Hill, 1978.

Jaffe D. Healing from within. New York: Alfred A. Knopf, Inc., 1980.

Joy of living library. Feel younger, live longer. New York: Rand McNally, 1977.

Jung CG. Man and his symbols. Garden City, New York: Doubleday, 1964.

Keys, A. Seven countries. Cambridge: Harvard University Press, 1980.

Kothari LK, Gupta OP. The yogic claim of voluntary control over the heart beat: an unusual demonstration. American Heart Journal. 1973; 86:282–4.

Lappé FM. Diet for a small planet. New York: Ballantine Books/ Random House, 1975.

Mann GV. A factor in yogurt which lowers cholesterolemia in man. Atherosclerosis. 1977; 26:335–40.

Mendeloff A. Dietary fiber and human health. New England Journal of Medicine. 1977; 297:811–14.

Miller NE, Dworkin BR. Effects of learning on visceral functions— biofeedback. New England Journal of Medicine. 1977; 297:1274.

Patel CH. Yoga and biofeedback in the management of stress in hypertensive patients. Clinical Science and Molecular Medicine. 1975; 48:171s–174s.

Patel CH, North WRS. Randomized controlled trial of yoga and biofeedback in the management of hypertension. Lancet. 1975; 2:93–5.

Patel CH. Reduction of serum cholesterol and blood pressure in hypertensive patients by behavior modification. J R. Coll Gen Pract. 1976; 26: 211–5.

Selected Bibliography

Pelletier KR. Mind as healer/mind as slayer. New York: Dell Publishing Company, 1977.

Peters RK, Benson H, Porter D. Daily relaxation response breaks in a working population. American Journal of Public Health. 1977; 67:946–53, 954–9.

Phillips RL, Lemon FR, Beeson WL, Kuzma JW. Coronary heart disease mortality among Seventh-Day Adventists with differing dietary habits. American Journal of Clinical Nutrition. 1978; 31:S191.

Pritikin N, McGrady P. Pritikin program for diet and exercise. New York: Grosset and Dunlap, 1979.

Richmond JB. Smoking and health: a report of the Surgeon General. Washington: U.S. Government Printing Office (017-000-00218-0), 1979.

Robertson D, Froelich JC, Carr RK, et al. Effects of caffeine on plasma renin activity, catecholamines and blood pressure. New England Journal of Medicine. 1978; 298:181–6.

Robertson JIS. Salt intake and the pathogenesis and treatment of hypertension. Clinical Science, 1979; 57:453s.

Robertson L, Flinders C, Godfrey B. Laurel's kitchen: a handbook for vegetarian cookery and nutrition. Petaluma, California: Nilgiri Press, 1976.

Sagon C. Pre-game meal: Cowboys show their oats. Dallas Times Herald, September 3, 1981, p. E1.

Samuels M, Samuels N. Seeing with the mind's eye. New York: Random House, 1975.

Satchidananda S. Integral yoga hatha. New York: Holt, Rinehart and Winston, 1970.

Scharffenberg JA. Problems with meat. Santa Barbara: Woodbridge Press, 1979.

Schwarz J. Voluntary controls. New York: E.P. Dutton, 1978.

Selye H. Stress without distress. New York: J.P. Lippincott Co., 1974.

Shapiro AP, Schwartz GE, Ferguson DCE, Redmond DP, Weiss SM. Behavioral methods in the treatment of hypertension: a review of their clinical status. Ann Intern Med. 1977; 86:626–36.

Shapiro AP, Benson H, Chobanian AV, et al. The role of stress in hypertension. Journal of Human Stress. 1979; 4:7–45.

Shekelle RB, Shyrock AM, Paul O, et al. Diet, serum cholesterol and death from coronary heart disease. The Western Electric Study. New England Journal of Medicine. 1981; 304:65–70.

Shulman M. The vegetarian feast. New York: Harper and Row, 1979.

Shulman M. Fast vegetarian feasts. New York: The Dial Press, 1981.

Selected Bibliography

Shurtless W, Aoyagi A. The book of tofu. Brookline: Autumn Press, 1975.

Sigler LH. Emotion and atherosclerotic heart disease. I. Electrocardiographic changes observed on the recall of past emotional disturbances. Brit J Med Psychol. 1967; 40:55–64.

Simpson HCR, Simpson RW, Lousley S, et al. A high carbohydrate leguminous diet improves all aspects of diabetic control. Lancet. 1981; i:1–7.

Southey P. The vegetarian gourmet cookbook. New York: Van Nostrand, 1980.

Stein H. Looking hard at number one. Esquire magazine. February 1981, pp. 20–1.

Stone RA, DeLeo J. Psychotherapeutic control of hypertension. New England Journal of Medicine. 1976; 294:80–4.

U.S. Select Committee on Nutrition and Human Needs. Dietary goals for the United States, 2nd ed. Washington: U.S. Government Printing Office (052-070-04376-8), 1977.

Weil AT. The marriage of the sun and moon. Boston: Houghton Mifflin, 1980.

Weil AT. The natural mind. Boston: Houghton Mifflin, 1973.

Wenger NK, Hellerstein HK (eds). Rehabilitation of the coronary patient. New York: John Wiley and Sons, 1978.

Wheatley D (ed). Stress and the heart. New York: Raven Press, 1977.

White AJ, Finn R. Meat induced hypercholesterolemia. Lancet. October 25, 1980, p. 922.

Witty H, Colchie ES. Better than store-bought. New York: Harper and Row, 1979.

Yagoda B. Getting psyched. Esquire magazine. April 1982, pp. 30–4.

Zurbel R, Zurbel V. The vegetarian family. New York: Prentice-Hall, 1978.

Index

Index